Care Management

Tasks and Workloads

Joan Orme

and

Bryan Glastonbury

MACMILLAN

First published 1993 by
THE MACMILLAN PRESS LTD
Houndmills, Basingstoke, Hampshire RG21 2XS
and London
Companies and representatives
throughout the world

ISBN 0–333–54409–9 hardcover
ISBN 0–333–54410–2 paperback

A catalogue record for this book is available
from the British Library.

11	10	9	8	7	6	5	4	3
03	02	01	00	99	98	97	96	95

Printed in Hong Kong

Series Standing Order (Practical Social Work)

If you would like to receive future titles in this series as they are published, you can
make use of our standing o⟩ ... To ... a standing order please contact your
bookseller or, in case of ⟨ ... us a⟩the address below with your name
and address and the name ⟩ of the series. Please st⟨te with which title you wish to
begin your standing order⟩. (If you live outside the ⟨nited Kingdom we may not have
the rights for your area, i⟩ ⟨ which case we will for⟨vard your order to the publisher
concerned.)

Customer Services Depart⟩ment, Macmillan Distribu⟨ion Ltd
Houndmills, Basingstoke, ⟩Hampshire RG21 2XS, En⟨land

To Geoff, Emily and Tim Orme,
who always manage to care

Contents

Acknowledgements

In preparing this text we have been aware that the requirements of good management systems are similar to those for good commentators. That is, those performing the management function or making the commentary need to be aware of the demands of the process, but sufficiently objective to be able to assess, modify and innovate. We are both academics, one with a background in policy and a passion for information technology, the other with a background in practice. Continuing study of workload management has meant that we have both been involved in research, consultancy and staff development work, especially in relation to the implementation of the National Health Service and Community Care Act, 1990. We recognised that what was lacking was someone with first hand practice experience in care management. In achieving the necessary objective, informed commentary, Georgiana Robertson has been an invaluable member of the team which produced this book. Her post as Assistant Coordinator, Community Care with Hampshire Social Services and her first-hand experience of setting up care management schemes for people with learning difficulties are excellent qualifications for involvement in the clarification of key concepts. Undertaking the reading of drafts, either jointly or individually, with vigilance and the practitioner's eye has made her an important part of the quality assurance of this volume. In many ways she has

xi

provided an excellent model of care management; however, if there are complaints from the consumer they should be directed at Joan Orme, whose capacity as editor in some ways equates with the service provider.

We would also like to acknowledge others who have contributed to the production of this text in a variety of ways. These include many colleagues at the University of Southampton and Hampshire Social Services who have provided the opportunity to share ideas. In particular we would like to thank Jon Clark, Sheena Glastonbury and Geoff Orme for their practical help in many different ways, and for their unswerving support and inspiration.

JOAN ORME
BRYAN GLASTONBURY

Introduction

Care management in community care is crucial for all those currently employed in the personal social services, but has particular relevance for professionally qualified social workers. Viewed positively it offers the opportunity to review practices and policies of service delivery, to be innovative and flexible, and to work more effectively with the consumers of the services. Viewed negatively it is a threat to the old order, the patterns of service delivery and, more significantly, employment. Will social workers simply change their title to care manager, or are there more fundamental changes required? In writing this book we are well aware of the concerns and we have set out to explore these and to clarify and codify some of the concepts that are around.

The profession of social work has been under threat for some time. The question of its survival was posed starkly by Brewer and Lait in 1980, although their questioning of the evidence on the efficacy of social work was not in itself effective. A greater challenge was posed by the Barclay Report (1982). It had been commissioned by the incoming Conservative Government, with a specific brief to analyse the role and functions of social workers. Implicit in the task, and at times explicit in the report, was the notion that social work did not have to be undertaken by large numbers of professionally qualified individuals. The concept of social

1

care planning carried with it suggestions that if social work was organised differently its functions could be carried out more effectively, drawing upon a variety of sources. The recommendations were made in a political climate which had as its aim the reduction of state intervention into the lives of individuals, while at the same time exercising more central control in areas of education, criminal justice, health service planning and the provision of social services. Other significant changes were introduced which had a direct impact on levels of service provision, for example limits on local authority spending, and a further report was commissioned. The Griffiths Report (1988) provided the seed of the idea of care management. It saw a role for local authorities in organising community care, but also introduced the notion that they should design and purchase, rather than be direct providers of, services. The speed at which these proposals were translated first into a White Paper (*Caring for People*, Department of Health, 1989) and then into legislation (Community Care and National Health Service Act 1990) demonstrates how they reflected the political will. The same speed, however, has disadvantaged the very individuals whose professional task will be directly affected by the proposed changes. There has been little opportunity for debate, for considered reflection or for resistance. Much activity has taken place at higher management levels, with regional discussions with health services and top-down exercises in producing community care plans. Local initiatives in the actual practice of planning, commissioning and implementing community care have had limited publicity, written either for an internal audience or in the specialist language of the academic researcher.

In commencing our task we discovered that writing about policy and legislation which is in the process of being implemented is fraught with difficulties. The first of these is that the subject itself is constantly being defined and redefined. When we commenced this text there was much rhetoric, but very little guidance on the implementation of policy. There was research, but little evidence that the findings could be easily translated into day-to-day practice by front line social workers. As we complete the text there are a growing number of policy documents and even practical guidelines emanating from the Department of Health and the Social Services Inspectorate. However they remain at the level of departmental activity and give no clues to the requirements and expectations of the role and task of front line social workers or their line managers. This is disappointing, but reassuring for us because it convinces us even more that this book needs to be written for those people whose roles and tasks in the provision of social services are clearly under scrutiny.

The second difficulty is a consequence of the process of definition and redefinition, and relates to the problems which arise when the terminology itself changes. In the early work in this country, and still in the United States the accepted term is *case management* and this term was at the core of the government thinking at the policy stages, as *Caring for People* illustrates. During the past months the generally used and now officially recognised term is *care management* (Department of Health, 1991a and b). The use of *care management* is significant because it is an acknowledgment that the work which will need to be done to ensure care in the community is not merely with an individual case, client or person but can involve the provision of a range of activities and services provided from a variety of sources. It is the package of care, involving whatever is necessary to enable the individual to continue living in the community, which will have to be managed, not the frequency and content of visits by a social worker to an individual client. The continued use of management is germane to our arguments because, while we acknowledge that in all social work tasks there are elements of management, the implications of current policy initiatives are that some recognition of the devolution of the management task is necessary. The fact that it is the *care* that will need to be managed and not the *case* is even more significant for us because of our firmly held belief that for any activity in social work to be managed there needs to be a recognition and overview of the work involved. That there is still the need for clear line management responsibility is reflected, for us, in the use of the term *service manager*. This identifies a first line management function with responsibility for the care managers but does not directly replace the team leader. We recognise that in some areas the title *service manager* has been used for those appointed to specific client groups or geographical areas, not always at the level of front line manager. However for our purposes the title does encompass what we feel are essential functions of a front line manager which are concerned with ensuring and assuring a service to consumers.

Such a debate highlights the fact that the legislation has brought with it changes in terminology which need definition and clarification, but, equally important, the need to be clear about what is meant by the use of terms with which social workers, and others, assume they are familiar. To assist understanding, and to clarify our usage of certain terms we have provided a glossary at the end of the book.

Care management has been defined in many ways, with much emphasis on the consumer orientation of the policy, and presumably the practice. It is about matching flexible services to identified needs rather than fitting people into inflexible services. This shift in emphasis is important in itself, but has significance for those who have had a crucial role in providing services. In considering this change we are conscious that stress has been put upon quality assurance and consumers, and we are in total agreement with Piachaud when he comments that 'The present Government has put all its emphasis on consumers and on management at the expense of providers of services and of professional standards; they have ignored the fact that professional autonomy is a major source not only of quality and service development but also of job satisfaction' (1991, p. 212). We would also argue that quality, service development and job satisfaction are obtained when the work of the front line social worker is properly managed.

In an earlier study of workload management (Glastonbury, Bradley and Orme, 1987) we maintained that there is a fundamental need for workload management schemes in social work. By this we mean that, at an individual level, a team level and an organisational level there needs to be an acknowledgement of the work that has to be done, the standard to which it must be done and the resources available to do it. In any workload management scheme there needs to be some notion of measurement, whether that is an actual measurement of how long it takes to do a particular task or a notional weighting of tasks in comparison to each other. This measurement is necessary to give a form of accounting for tasks in order to ascertain what is 'enough' for individual workers and what constitutes parity between the workloads of individuals. We recognise that to implement such schemes can be perceived as managerial interference in the autonomy of individual workers, but argue that, properly handled, such schemes are more likely to give protection to workers and, properly calculated, they help to ensure that workers are given the appropriate time to carry out the tasks expected of them to best professional standards. This helps to promote job satisfaction on the part of the worker and also assures quality for the consumer.

Our task in this text is therefore to clarify the implication of care management for those who are currently employed as front line social workers. In attempting this we have identified three overarching themes which help to divide the book into sections. The first theme is whether the implementation of care management will in fact constitute a change in the work that social workers undertake with individual clients. In the first three chapters of the book we address the way in which care management can be perceived as a continuation of policy, philosophy and practice of themes which have their roots in the Seebohm Report, if not the report on the Poor Law! In a largely theoretical way we explore such continuities in the light of current criticisms of social work practice and seek to show how care management can offer opportunities for addressing, for example, anti-discriminatory practice. The second theme is the implications for social workers of the tasks involved in care management. This includes an analysis of the possible organisation of service delivery and, critically, the professional background, qualification and management status of those performing the tasks. Chapters 4 and 5 are focused on practice and give detailed accounts of the requirements of care management and the possible ways in which it can be organised. In these accounts we are constantly aware that ultimately for schemes to be implemented they will need to be translated into appropriate workloads for the front line workers. This is the third theme, which is explored in Chapters 6 and 7. These chapters also provide a summary of our main arguments. In Chapter 6 we present a framework for good care management which leads us, in Chapter 7, to give guidelines for the particular workload concerns of care management.

We have set out to write a text which will inform those at the front line of the social work profession of some of the thinking behind the changes brought about by the implementation of care management in community care, but more particularly the implications for them as professionally qualified workers and the possible changes which will be required. It is not a text on how to do it, a users' manual. It is a text which will alert students, workers and front line managers to the concepts and issues, but more particularly the possible consequences of community care for themselves and for the individuals, families and groups about whom, and for whom, they care.

1

Community Care, Care Management and Workload Management

Different nations, different cultures, develop their own philosophies of welfare. In North America there is a prevailing current of self-dependence, reinforced by the supportive values of the many immigrant cultures which make up its population. National and state participation in social services is well established in appreciation of the fact that wholly private or voluntary systems will not meet the needs of less privileged citizens in a comprehensive fashion. Yet the public services do not dominate, either in size or influence, and the resulting social services mix is a lucky dip. On the up side there is enormous variety, in size, policy, organisational structure and method of working, so that America is a test-bed for new ideas, for pushing forward new ways of helping people. On the down side the services available to a particular individual in a particular locality may be comprehensive and progressive, but just as likely may be patchy and eccentric.

In contrast Britain, while practising a mixed economy in offering social services, has a long commitment to public provision and, despite some wavering, has moved gradually to accept the dominance of the public sector. For many decades Britain has maintained a standardised range of services, usually organised on a local basis, but running

7

according to national legislation and central government policy. The down side may be the lack of variety. The up side includes a capacity to take a nationwide approach, to review and set policies through a broadly based planned route, and to assess the overall state of affairs from moral, political, economic and 'best practice' angles.

Despite the seeming consistency of this approach, British social history is littered with major reviews of the social services, some of which have led to fundamental change, while others gather dust in a forgotten corner. A century and a half ago there was a review and major restructuring of the social services departments of the day, operated under the Poor Law. Community care, known then as domiciliary, parish or outdoor relief, was becoming too expensive, so was banned for all except those with serious mental or physical defects. This is not to say that helping a family in the community was necessarily more costly than residential provision (it was not!), but there were economic and moral doubts about such an approach. The economic problem stemmed from the fact that community help was more attractive to the population, so many more eligible people had the temerity to apply for it, and the overall bill became burdensome. The moral aspect had two elements. There was concern that people given outdoor relief might achieve a standard of living with state help which others could not reach through their own efforts; and there was a feeling that state benefits should only be provided in a way which was unpleasant enough to put off all but the most desperate.

The solution was residential care, coupled with the transfer of Poor Law administration from local parish officials (too many of whom were considered to be a soft touch) to a more centralised authority. The core provision was to be the workhouse, operating a regime which would make anyone think twice before seeking a place. There was compulsory hard labour for all able-bodied residents: 'You have got to find work which anybody can do, and which nearly everybody dislikes doing [otherwise] you will have your workhouse crowded up with loafers' (J. S. Davy, Principal Officer of the Poor Law Division of the Local Government Board in evidence to the Royal Commission, 1905–9). The worst material living standards were ensured by contracting out the responsibilities for operating workhouses to the lowest tender.

From our viewpoint in the 1990s, has anything altered, other than the view held in some circles that community rather than residential care will work more effectively, be cheaper, and meet prevailing moral standpoints? Certainly many of the core issues remain in the forefront, like the continuing search for the least expensive way to provide for needy people, reassessing the interface of state and self-help, devising means tests and obstacles in order to keep down the level of demand, and striving to keep some control over the extent and nature of service provision. Also we seem not to have lost our commitment, despite the evidence of our own experiences, to the view that organisational restructuring, rather than consolidation and refinement, is the route to achieving change.

At the same time there have been fundamental changes, not least to Britain's basic democratic system. The 1834 Royal Commission addressed itself to a Parliament which represented a narrowly defined and privileged section of society. All women and most working people, including customers of the personal social services, lacked the power of the vote. Since then, as political rights have spread, so has sensitivity to the views of the wider society. New concepts have come into circulation, like that of public participation in decision making about services, or the view that those whose circumstances oblige them to make use of our welfare provisions have as much right to courtesy and fairness as any other citizen. The process of reviewing how 'democratic' or how 'right' we are as a society is a continuing one. At present the focus is on aspects of discrimination on the basis of gender and race. The overarching notion is that of consumerism, defined in terms of the rights and powers of all consumers, the choices they are offered and the way they are treated. Carlyle would find little present-day support (in public at least!) for the domineering paternalism of his view that 'If paupers are made miserable, paupers will needs decline in multitude. It is a secret known to all rat-catchers' (Carlyle, 1839).

Another realisation which has made us more considerate towards people with needs is that inferred by the idea of rehabilitation. Early Victorians accepted the traditional view that some people who had 'slipped' could find their feet again, and become accepted and productive members of society. However there was also the opinion that quite a large minority, a 'submerged tenth' perhaps, could be written off. Common humanity might require that they be given minimal help to stretch out a miserable existence, but they would continue to be a burden on society. Later Victorians, ranging from Octavia Hill, with her practical demonstrations of the impact of sensitive housing management, to Herbert Gladstone, arguing that criminals could do something more useful and less soul destroying than spend their days on a treadmill, began to challenge prevailing attitudes. Beatrice and Sidney Webb took up the cause, and now the idea of rehabilitative, remedial and supportive services to help people live as near as possible independent lives within society has become part of the bedrock of social policy.

Community care

This happy combination of sound economics (rehabilitated people can be productive, and may not need continuing support) and common humanity (people are happier living in their own homes or, at least, doing something useful) is central to the motivation which has turned us away from dependence on residential care towards community-based solutions to people's problems. The switch is not new or sudden, but has come about gradually, so that there has been time both to strengthen the commitment to community care as the most suitable way forward and to identify some of the difficulties which such an approach has to tackle.

The real difficulty faced at the start of the last century was the relative attractiveness of outdoor relief, and the level of demand this engendered. The solution of the time reflected the choice of an approach (residential warehousing without anything recognisable as treatment) which was simple to administer and susceptible to closer control. The problem of high levels of need remains, but now there is no longer a simple or cost-saving solution. Warehousing is neither morally acceptable (though it still exists for some clients), nor does it contribute towards rehabilitation. It is many years since the Webbs (1929) argued that specialised needs demanded equally specialised services, if the policy of helping people back to independent living was to work. Since then we have discovered that incorporating specialisation and treatment into residential provisions is both very expensive and often unsuited to the task in hand. There is a compelling contradiction in seeking to enable community living by taking people out of the community. While it is acknowledged that there are at times unavoidable circumstances that require removal from the community, there has been a growing acknowledgement that care needs to be in the community.

For the 1990s the agenda seems to be set. 'Community care means providing the services and support which people who are affected by problems of ageing, mental illness, mental handicap or physical or sensory disability need to be able to live as independently as possible in their own homes, or in "homely" settings in the community. The Government is firmly committed to a policy of community care which enables such people to achieve their full potential' (Department of Health, 1989, para.1.1). This is scarcely a novel statement. It repeats what has been policy for many years.

Similar approaches, though with restrictive conditions, apply to other client groups. Children are preferably cared for in the community, if possible by their own parent(s), but this has to be conditional on a thorough assessment and continuing monitoring of any risk to which the child might be subjected. Helping offenders in the community is also advocated, using probation or community service orders, this time dependent on the severity of the offence, the offender's record and the risk to the community. The Health Service, albeit under pressure from shortage of funds as much as through a philosophical commitment, has sought to minimise dependence on long stays in hospital for those with chronic illness.

Providing care in the community is thus widely accepted and broadly based. The controversial issue in this context is not so much about care in the community as about the pressure for care by the community. The view that communities should take responsibility for the care of their own needy people has a long history (nearly half a millennium ago parishes took care of their own paupers), but has weakened as circumstances have changed. The growth of industrial society, urbanisation, the erosion of the extended family, and labour mobility have all played a part. So has the increasing proportion of dependent people who survive in any modern community. Alongside these changes a view has grown up that, in relation to certain needy groups, including children at risk, people with physical disabilities or learning difficulties and dependent elderly people, the state (or local authority) should have a central role.

In contrast there have been vocal expressions of opinion that, as a nation, we are too dependent, and should be more determined to stand on our own feet or get on our own bicycles. For the personal social services these opinions were given more precision in the Barclay Report (1982), with the view that social workers, to be called community social workers, should turn partly away from direct provision towards enabling local community networks to meet needs. The Report was shelved, and an authoritative analysis of community networks (Allan, 1983) cast doubts on their potential for the task, or indeed whether such networks really existed. Nevertheless failure to take real notice of the importance of the relationship between local authority service agencies and local populations, especially at a time when resources are not keeping up with the growth in needs, has damaging effects. People cannot get statutory help, lack strong enough networks to spread the load of their needs, and become dependent on individuals. By the start of the 1990s we were faced with vast numbers of informal helpers–carers of elderly people, parents of severely handicapped children, and others – who were themselves trying to cope with intolerable stress. In other contexts we have become increasingly aware of situations where people are outside the span of mainstream helping networks, and often of public services as well. Ethnic minorities are an example, forced by practical problems (like language differences), or cultural misunderstandings, or straight racial discrimination into a degree of self-dependence well beyond anything expected of the indigenous population.

In asserting the primacy of community care, *Caring for People* (Department of Health, 1989) took up the issue in a mixed welfare economy. It attempted a balance between in-puts from the community, the voluntary and private sectors, and public services. It confirmed the role of local communities as major providers in time of need, although with specific responsibility placed on local authorities for en-suring that carers are assisted and supported (para.2.3). More significantly the framework of providers of services is extended to incorporate the independent sector, an amal-gamation of local networks, local voluntary and private organisations, and, potentially, large private personal social service corporations.

The leading role of the local authority has been con-firmed, but less as the direct service provider and more as an impresario, assessing needs, identifying relevant services, arranging who will provide the services, where necessary purchasing them, monitoring progress and quality, and re-viewing outcomes. The message for the 1990s is that the state will oversee community care, as well as residential care, but may reduce its part as a direct provider.

Managing community care

Nevertheless the thrust of the second half of the twentieth century has been towards treatment services in the community, albeit more slowly than many would wish. This in turn has exposed problems of service management, in particular factors which promote administrative complexity. Community care is characterised by diversity, whether of the domestic circumstances of clients or of the specialised range of services needed to help them. Managing diversity calls on skills which were scarcely recognised in the Victorian workhouse, such as setting priorities, balancing workloads, operating multi-disciplinary teamwork and respecting client rights. The complexity is apparent at senior agency level, where there has to be awareness of the cost and potential benefits of a wide range of service approaches; and in the service front line, where diverse workloads have to be received, allocated and held by a mixed staff group. The management of community care has been made still more challenging by the simultaneous process of closing down many residential facilities, and so pushing into the community accumulated generations of clients needing new services.

As well as diversity in the needs and range of client contexts, managerial complexity has been increased by a steady flow of different forms of treatment and ways of implementing them. It is not relevant to enter into debate here about the content of treatment methods, but some observations are pertinent. Social work and linked professions have put forward great variety in what they have to offer, but the impact has not been entirely beneficial. The lack of agreement or lack of evidence about which intervention methods are the most useful has taken some authority away from the views of service professionals. This in turn has confused senior managers, who are themselves under pressure to enforce cost-effective management systems which have the result of favouring some approaches (usually the shorter and cheaper ones) rather than others. More fundamentally, staff in front line servicing have various reasons for keeping open a range of treatment options, such as the desire to use methods which suit their own aptitudes, to allow more subtlety in the development of treatment plans, or to give clients more choice. This poses difficult problems for workload management systems. The individual worker, responsible for self-management, needs to ask, 'How can I have the maximum beneficial impact on a client without the intervention becoming too time consuming?' Managers, with responsibility for allocation and ensuring service delivery, have to pose questions such as 'Can a social worker who prefers a more time consuming approach to clients use this as grounds for carrying a smaller caseload than other workers?'

The combination of diversity in client contexts with variety in treatment methods has crowded the scene. In the first instance, workload management and self-management become complex matters. Going further, the knowledge base required by staff has expanded, whether it is knowledge of law, local circumstances, therapeutic techniques, or a range of topics on which they need to be informed. An additional and newer area of complexity has its origins in the issue of balancing state (public) with self or community help for needy clients. The Victorians had an explicit distinction between undeserving people (those who were to blame for their plight) and the deserving (blameless), who were to get a better standard of service, generally from a voluntary organisation. The extent to which people had tried to help themselves influenced their moral categorisation, and the pressure for self-help was maintained by the deterrents built into seeking other, especially Poor Law, help. Collectivist philosophies (such as socialism) have emerged to challenge this approach to the less fortunate section of society, but rulers with inclinations to extol the virtues of individualism have dominated British governments, so the basic pattern has remained, though an assessment of severity of need now sits beside or has replaced a moral judgement. If you have a problem look to your own resources, or those of your family and friends, to help you through it; if that fails then seek help through local networks and voluntary groups; only if that too is no use, try to get state support.

This approach is underpinned by a clear and widely understood hierarchy of priorities. There is also, arguably, a logic to the sequence, because in theory it ensures that those who can help themselves or get local aid do so, and only the most severe needs command state provision. The description of what is severe can be modified from time to time, to respond to changes in resource levels or public attitudes. For example, 'severe' in this context can be interpreted as a lack of support systems rather than the extent of a disability or learning difficulty. Hence, recent government policies, most obviously in *Caring for People* (Department of Health, 1989), have sought to impose a new categorisation. While reasserting the commitment to community care, the idea of a gradation of needs, with the most severe being provided for by the statutory agency, is replaced by procedures based on the notion of supply-side competition. Needs which are assessed as serious enough to warrant service provision are met by one provider – or a combination of providers – using predetermined intervention methods and contracted primarily according to cost (for a given quality).

Care management

The government's preferred method both for achieving these changes and for enhancing the whole framework of community care, is care or case management. Well before the concept was taken up at government level, Renshaw defined it as follows: 'A case management system is usually one in which the provision of services to meet the needs of individual clients is the responsibility of one agency or worker. The services themselves may be provided by different agencies but the case manager coordinates the services and ensures that needs are met' (Renshaw, 1988).

Case management has its origins in the USA in the early 1970s. Faced with problems of organisational fragmentation and the need for better co-ordination, the USA had a set of problems similar to those which led to the formation of the Seebohm Committee (1968). However there was too much diversity of agency control and ownership to permit a British-type solution (that is, the formation of unitary social services departments). Parts of the USA, therefore, looked to those who came to be labelled 'case managers' to plan, overview and co-ordinate work with clients. These developments were not confined to specific client groups, though they tended to be most necessary (and effective) for long term clients. Much American case management is heavily involved with the accountancy/budgetary aspects of case activity, often in circumstances where a service funding agency uses a case manager to co-ordinate and oversee the use of its funds by service providing agencies. The first use of the label and some of the processes in the UK is generally associated with Kent Social Services Department (Challis and Davies, 1986). In the discussions immediately following the publication of *Caring for People* (Department of Health, 1989) the term 'case manager' was used. However as the debate has gone on the official publications have used 'care manager'. In view of this, and for the reasons identified in our introduction, we will use 'care manager' during the rest of this text.

It is too simplistic to view care management just as a route to diversifying the provision of services, or as a form of monitoring and controlling the use of resources. So what is it? A suitable starting-point is to describe the role and tasks of the care manager. The label itself may be relatively new in Britain, but much of the concept is not. A care manager may well operate in part very much like our current understanding of a key worker. The primary role of the key worker is to take responsibility for the co-ordination of work with a client. A key worker is assigned to a case when there are service inputs from several staff, possibly from more than one agency, so that there is a need to ensure that the 'inputs' gel into a coherent service for the client, that communication amongst staff and with the client is maintained, and that opportunities exist for reviewing the situation and making further plans. In short the minimal task of a key worker is to enable the staff working with the client to function as a team.

The role of the key worker can and often does go further, depending very much on the level of available authority. In some situations the key worker is seeking to co-ordinate a service plan fixed at a meeting (such as a case conference) or prescribed by a more senior member of staff: but on other occasions s/he has the responsibility for drawing up the plan and negotiating the parts played by the rest of the team. Occasionally key workers also have direct decision-making control over some resources, though more often they endure the frustration of lacking such authority. Indeed, though key workers are often social workers, they can also be residential or day care officers, community psychiatric nurses or community mental health nurses. Whatever their background they are rarely at a senior level in their organisation.

The care manager's role has some similarity to that of the key worker, and issues about control of resources and staff are shared. However care management builds on the key worker concept in terms both of task and of process. Several new tasks are involved. One has to do with costing the service to be offered to a client, with a view both to relating this cost to the resources allocated to the client and to contributing to a wider workload accountancy system. The objectives of this approach are to get away from the traditional practices of offering open-ended service, and of accounting for a commitment to a client in terms of a service rather than a calculable financial liability. Instead, the assessment of the client's needs will lead, via a priority rating and care plan, into a statement of the funds to be attached to meeting those needs. Once a care management system is fully operational it will be possible to work out what services those funds will purchase, whether from the statutory agency or some other source, and where the best prices are on offer. A 'package of care' will then be determined between care manager and client, based initially on the needs identified in the assessment, but ultimately on the resources available to pay for the package. Depending on the model in operation the manager may be solely the purchaser of the care package, or additionally involved as a service provider.

Another new task relates to using the independent sector. If this sector does not exist in any adequate sense (a likely position in many areas), then there will be an initial developmental role. The job of working with an independent sector is concerned with keeping in touch with what it can offer, inviting tenders, commissioning services, negotiating service contracts, monitoring to ensure contracts are observed and checking the quality of provisions. Tenders and contracts require specialised, including legal knowledge, so it is likely that the care manager will not have to do this work, or will get professional help with it. Quality control is another task which may be handled separately, perhaps through a quality control unit in the local authority.

We have already seen that care managers are at the hub of the care management system, but they may well not be the only staff involved. The care manager may be sharing the provision of a service to the client with others, or contracting it out entirely. Someone (often called a broker) may be in the team as a resource raiser or developer, and a carer or advocate may take part to represent the interests of the client. A role division is also likely between a care manager, who carries responsibility for specified clients, and a more senior member of staff (we call her/him a service manager) who has an overview of clients in a particular group or location. If the care manager is a social worker, then the service manager may fill a role comparable to that of team leader, that is the manager of the care manager.

Care and workload management

Despite this outline of the role and tasks of care managers and their support staff, it still remains valid to look again at the question, 'What is care management?' and seek a different type of response. Is it a method of social work or social service? Or is it a form and style of service management? The answer to both questions is probably 'yes'. Care management is both a form of social work and social service in the sense that it is about ways of working with and relating to clients, about client involvement and choice, and about service planning and delivery. At the same time care management is a technique for organising a package of care for a client, in response to the needs identified in the assessment and service availability. Its viability in this context, therefore, should be viewed in the light of its fit with wider agency management frameworks, and with prevailing approaches to field level workload management.

To understand more clearly the relevance of this assertion, a summary of front line workload management might be helpful (for a more detailed discussion see Glastonbury, Bradley and Orme, 1987). The raw materials of workload management are the tasks of staff, mainly social workers, in the personal social services. For them a workload is made up of cases (combining into a caseload) plus a range of additional jobs, such as intake, office duties and training. The caseload itself may be made up of a mixture of client types, some to be handled in future through care management, some by other approaches.

Workload management is about the systematic handling of cases and other components of the workload, an evaluation (usually a weighting) of the various pieces of work to enable them to be related to a workload ceiling or working week, a further evaluation (qualitative) to check the balance of the workload and its fit with the skills and interests of the worker, and a supervisory process which tracks a piece of work from start to finish. For a front line manager (or a self-managing senior practitioner or outposted worker) there are the additional tasks of scrutinising referrals, giving them a priority rating, allocating them to staff, balancing the workloads of a team, and operating a routine to deal with emergencies or important work which arrives at a time when all staff are functioning at the workload ceiling.

The objectives of a comprehensive workload management system include ensuring that the best available service is offered to needy clients, operating a fair rationing process when that is necessary, seeking service approaches which maximise cost-effectiveness, protecting and developing staff by confirming that they have a suitable workload both in nature and volume, and keeping the turnover of work on as even a path as possible.

Narrowing down to the management of work with clients, the overarching managerial concept is turnover, which takes in the three stages of opening cases, providing services, and reviewing cases. For care management the contents of each sequence are set out in Table 1.1.

For both the professional worker and the service manager there is a continuous process of comparing the importance and progress of this sequence between different cases and with other kinds of work. If pressures from elsewhere become too intense, then delaying or postponement devices have to come into play: if pressures ease, then processes can be speeded up or other tasks taken on. All of these activities require judgement and information. The judgement is professional and managerial, to ensure that basic objectives are not lost. It is important to keep in mind that these workloads are not being managed in a haven of tranquillity with plenty of time for reflection, but in the hiatus of an office being bombarded with demands which are neither evenly phased nor predictable. The information required is detailed up-to-

Table 1.1   *Sequences of care management: workload implications*

Opening cases	Identifying need
	Referral and filtering
	Assessment
	Formulating care plan
	Priority rating/rationing
	Costings/funding decision
	Care package negotiation
Service provision	*(a) Purchaser role*
	Planning care package implementation
	Care package specifications
	Invitations to tender and/or searching for service providers
	Contracting tasks
	(b) Provider role
	Supplying services
	Overseeing and co-ordinating servicing
	Quality checking
	Interim or end of service review
Reviewing cases	Evaluation of impact of care package
	Reassessment if needed
	Termination of care management
	Termination of contract with provider and placed with another provider
	Case closure

date material about clients and resources, preferably on screen in response to a few keyboard strokes. Often it is needed very quickly, especially if there are any risk factors that need to be picked out. In a care management system, as we shall see in later chapters, new ranges of information are needed, most significantly a catalogue of services, service providers, quality ratings, charges and budget monitoring.

Some of the proposed or perceived adjuncts to care management seem set to increase workload pressures. One is establishing a right to assessment. This could mean that assessing a new client has to be given priority over providing service, regardless of professional views about the relative urgency or severity of the circumstances. Another is the desire to incorporate consumerist values, to allow time and opportunity for clients (or their advocates) to help in the assessment of needs and planning services.

If care management is to operate effectively it needs workload management. Experience suggests that some basic guidelines ought to be followed. In a previous study (1987, pp. 182–3) we listed 19 practical points. We shall draw on them in Chapter 7, when we seek to suggest a working model of workload management for care management. The next two chapters pursue some of the contentious issues touched on so far. They provide an examination of some of the key concepts and an evaluation of the changes that they might, or might not, initiate.

Summary

This chapter has plotted the evolution of care management. It has argued that the concept of community care has been with us for some time and that the emergence of care management, while being in some ways a logical extension of community care, also raises many new issues. The first is that care management involves care by the community as well as care in the community. Second, within the context of a mixed economy of welfare provision the distinction between public and private provision underpins a debate about the tension between quality and cost. In introducing some of the terms and concepts embedded within care management in community care we begin to seek clarification of what needs to be done, who will do it and how it will be organised and managed. We indicate that the complexity of the process has implications for the tasks that have to be performed by front line staff and that workload management is a basic prerequisite for the protection of the worker and the assurance of quality. Before expanding on this theme it is necessary to look at some of the other issues surrounding care management, the resistances and the criticisms.

2

Issues in Care Management

Introduction

Having considered the evolution of the thinking behind care management in community care it is important to document the responses. The prospect of care management has provoked a range of comments from practitioners, many critical. Remarks made to us include (of American case management): 'It's really just project management: it's got nothing to do with professional practice' and (of Kent's scheme): 'It reduces the importance of social work values, and means that they can now use untrained people to do what used to be done by social workers.' The gist of some comments is that care management is an American import, picked up by the government and trendy right-wing local authorities. A widespread implication is that whatever the USA has to offer about professional social work it has badly organised social work services which should not be a model for Britain and only attract the government because of the role played in them by the private and non-profit sectors of the economy. Others, albeit a minority, do seem to feel that there is a tendency to inflexible bureaucratic behaviour in the current domination of social services departments, which might be eased by measures to loosen monopoly and increase choice.

Comments about care management from within social

services departments' front line teams, like 'It's a cheat, a device for cutting public spending on social work' and 'There's nothing new about it. We've been doing all these care package things for years', continue the negative trend. Overall there is deep suspicion about care management, focused on three criticisms:

1. The idea that care management is dominated by budgetary and resource matters, and represents the first stage of taking the personal social services out of the welfare state.
2. The view that although the language has changed, in substance there is nothing new about care management.
3. The feeling that social work will diminish in importance, leaving clients to be helped by less skilled people, and causing a major upheaval in professional staffing.

The intention of this chapter is to identify some of the issues which arise under the first of these criticisms and to look at significant themes within it. The first concerns how far care management leads to a devolution of resources and decision making to the front line, specifically to the purchaser/provider/consumer interface. Following on from the discussion of devolution it is necessary to question whether devolution will reach through to the customers of the services. Does care management offer a genuine opportunity to incorporate consumerist interests, or is it just hype?

The second criticism, that there is nothing new about care management, will be dealt with in Chapter 3, where we will explore both the continuities of, and the challenges for, social work practice. These have to inform the way that we respond to the third criticism, which is based on the concern that care management will alter the make-up of front line workers, for the most part making them less well qualified. Are there justifiable fears that this will lead to a deterioration in service? These issues, while introduced here, will be explored in a detailed examination of the care management process in Chapter 4.

Whether the authors' and readers' personal standpoint is for or against these proposed developments, most of us can probably agree that the clients for whom they are intended in the first instance, people who are elderly, or with mental illness, learning difficulties or disabilities, are not well served under existing arrangements or by existing levels of resources. The intention of the following chapters is to encourage front line workers to work creatively with the opportunities offered by policy changes and seek to improve the services available.

Care management and resources

The accusation that care management is a resource-led system raises a number of issues. What is meant by the notion of a resource-led system, and is it intrinsically a bad thing? Where will the necessary resources come from? What sorts of budgetary procedures will be needed? To make sense of what is proposed about resource matters it is necessary to distinguish between procedures which are an essential part of the care management process and those which feature because they are considered desirable, perhaps for political reasons. Integral to care management is the attempt to bring into personal social services planning and delivery a form of accountancy which makes it easier to monitor and control the use of scarce resources. That is, procedures are being introduced which allow the care manager (usually a social worker) and the agency to know from the start of a contact with a client the full cost of the services which are under consideration. In some circumstances, such as a proposal to place a person with learning difficulties and challenging behaviour in a residential setting outside the local authority, such costing is already necessary in order to get approval to place. Care management seeks to extend the costing process into areas which are rarely quantified at present. Our contention is that items such as workers' time, whether they be social worker, home carer or occupational therapist, should be included in the calculations of the cost of the service delivery. Working out costs and setting charges is one of the major new information needs which will be picked up later in the book.

Attached to the government's care management plans are two further resource measures which are not in themselves a necessary part of a care management system, but which at the start of the 1990s have political support. They are, firstly, that services to implement care packages should not be taken solely from within the statutory sector (though such an arrangement would have been perfectly feasible), but should be taken, where possible, from the independent sector. As we shall see later, this appears to broaden the base from which services can be drawn, but could have the opposite effect if local authority provision declines in areas where the independent sector does not show itself capable of playing a full part.

The second measure concerns raising resources to supplement public funding. This would be consistent with government policies throughout the 1980s, where there may have been a theoretical commitment to greater privatisation, but a practice of segmented privatisation coupled to pressure to seek top up funding for minimal public grants. This has occurred extensively in education (schools and universities) and health, so it is hardly surprising that it now finds its way into the personal social services.

Does this warrant the label 'resource-led system'? The authors of the White Paper, *Caring for People*, might prefer a categorical denial. For them care management is led by a sequence which starts with a thorough assessment, available as a right, and follows through into a package of care, negotiated with the client. The process is supported by measures to ensure acceptable quality and deal with customer complaints, and reinforced by the expectation that the assessment will be free-standing, needs-based, uncontaminated by a consideration of what services are or are not available in practice.

If this view raises howls of disbelief, it is in part because service staff have always expected to operate a compromise between what a client needs and what can be offered. The inadequacy of resources to meet needs is a permanent state of affairs in the personal social services. In this sense care management is as resource-led as its predecessors, and to accept such reality is reasonable and sensible. However it is important to see the validity of a distinction between the volume and nature of resources. There is a context to the debate about the volume of service resources. Part of it is the fact that national expenditure on personal social services has increased in real terms in the last decade by about a third, though arguably to be more than swallowed up by increases in the number of people with illness, disabilities and other needs. Another part of the context is that some client groups, including people who are elderly or in some way disabled, are regularly pushed to the back, behind children, in the queue for scarce resources.

Superimposed on this difficult morale-sapping reality is the knowledge that substantial funds pumped into helping needy people through the National Health Service and the Department of Social Security are being withdrawn. People with mental illness and learning difficulties are being pushed out of health care as hospitals are closed. Social security payments for residential care are being reduced, and are to be phased out. If social services departments, either alone or in partnership with the independent sector, are to take over responsibility for these clients, will these resources now be made available to fund packages of care?

There is no answer to this core question. In postponing the full implementation of the NHS and Community Care Act the government of the day acknowledged that a cost existed, and decided that the funds could not be found. In the past some portion of the shortfall would have been met by increased funds from local government sources. Throughout the 1980s, as direct central government support for local government fell, the local authorities themselves sought, often with success, to protect the personal social services. Again there is obscurity about the possibilities for the 1990s, given the long-running hiatus over the system for local government revenue, but the signs are that central government controls will reduce local flexibility.

Is there any other source for resources? Undoubtedly some people have looked hopefully to the independent sector, perhaps with an image in mind of the structure of non-profit organisations and trusts which makes such an impact across the Atlantic. Imaginations have run wild, ranging from suggestions of a national lottery to views of social workers rattling collection tins outside the local shopping precinct or running jumble sales. All that can be said with any certainty is that the British independent sector is many years, if not decades, away from being in a position to make a significantly greater impact on resource levels, and that the scale of resource needs is in a different league compared to the potential contribution from non-governmental sources.

As argued earlier, concern with resources is not solely about quantity. It is also about their nature and quality. It is hard to be anything but cynical about the idea that care management and the promotion of an independent sector will improve the supply of resources. Indeed the extra workload in the system (as will be discussed later) is a probable additional cost. However it can be argued that the separation of client assessment from an awareness of available resources (or should one say 'known shortages'?) will promote a more imaginative and flexible view of people's needs and how they can be met. Knowledge of shortages, that there are no vacancies in the day centre, no free home helps, no specialised therapeutic facilities, does seem likely to sap the enthusiasm and creativity of any worker carrying out an assessment. In one sense a free spirit, an imagination guided by good training, but unfettered by knowledge of reality round the corner, is a cruel exploitation of a client. Why raise a client's hopes with a superbly creative assessment, only to have to follow up with a postscript to the effect that of course none of these proposed services are actually available? In another sense, and this is what *Caring for People* wishes to pursue, there is the chance that new ideas in the assessment will stimulate the development of new types of service. Perhaps these new ideas will be a spur to action within social services departments, but more probably (at least in a Conservative Government's eyes) they will stir up the independent sector. Local volunteers and voluntary groups will see exciting opportunities to be helpful; non-profit organisations will discover new directions; entrepreneurs will see scope for new markets.

Whether such aspirations are real possibilities or flights of fancy, one reality remains. Knowledge of shortages and inadequacies in service resources is a dead weight. It does impede a free ranging and creative assessment. The challenge to social workers, and one of the most difficult tasks in care management, is to achieve a balance, to work with the client on developments which are imaginative, but which are also realistic and do not raise false hopes.

Budgetary procedures

Turning from global issues of resources, and from arguments about ways to increase variety, flexibility and creativity, there remain more mundane concerns about the sorts of budgetary procedures which will be needed to operate care management. It is possible to see how this works by tracking through the sequences of care management in Table 2.1. The left-hand column indicates the activity associated with care management, while the right-hand column catalogues the associated resource needs and activities.

This view of the way budgetary processes interact with client work covers both internal and (theoretically optional) external situations. For the internal process it is clear that there is a need for extensive new information on client needs and means as well as services, plus a procedure for costing

Table 2.1 *Sequences of care management: budgetary implications*

Activity	Resource element
Action prior to dealing with a referral	Source book or computer database of information setting out prices, locations, availability, features and quality of all available services.
Assessment of needs and means test for eligibility	Ability to inform client of services available, with cost and any payment implications for client; format for means testing client
Priority rating of client needs and decision about resource (funding) ceiling from public sources	Costings of services as before, plus information on funds/services available for allocation for a given priority level, taking into account means test results
Negotiation of care package	Costs related to direct provision and external purchasing or contracting; resource earmarked for fund-raising effort; procedures for client contribution
Ordering direct provision and contracting or purchasing external provision; arranging or liaising with broker about resource raising effort	Tendering and contracting procedures. Charitable and other sources of funds. opportunities for fund or other resource raising (brokerage activity)
Overseeing service provision and monitoring outcomes	Standard income and expenditure book-keeping; accessible performance indicators and cost–benefit checks
Review and closure of case	Procedures for handling over-or under-spending, or for considering further service provision
Post closure	Incorporating case income and expenditure into overall team or area or agency accounts

and pricing services and/or the costs themselves, and a book-keeping facility. If the independent sector is added, then there is the need for specialised knowledge and procedures for business interactions with different types of private or voluntary group, both in the context of contracting for services and in monitoring service outputs. Resource generating involves still more information and activity.

It is equally clear that care management, because of the introduction of these budgetary measures, is likely to demand a heavy staff involvement. The extra workload in providing information and carrying through the range of resource calculations will be substantial, leading either to much reduced caseloads for social workers as care managers (assuming they take on the extra tasks) or to the need for new support staff, or to the use of existing support staff in different ways. The extra workload also requires new skills in areas which are not traditionally part of training syllabi for service personnel, although they have been part of the repertoire of administrative staff.

The accountancy aspects of care management require fundamental changes in the way social services departments typically handle expenditures and the associated book-keeping. The usual model is that funds are allocated by the local authority to the social services department, and organised under a range of staffing and non-staffing budgetary categories to meet different sorts of costs. There are categories for different types of staff, for computers and furniture, for building maintenance, and many others. The total number of budgetary categories (or 'heads') is likely to run into several hundreds. Budgetary accountability is then handled by keeping a close check on claims made on each category, to ensure that each claim is valid, to monitor the spacing of expenditure as the financial year passes, and to make certain that there is no over-spending, or if that is not possible, to know exactly where over-spending occurred. In short this complex system of budgetary categories and procedures, which will be in the hands of designated finance staff, provides the guarantee that books are balanced, money goes where it is intended, and everything is legitimate.

Very little of this budgetary process touches social workers directly. They may be able to make an allocation of small resources to certain clients, and will routinely apply for approval of cost-carrying decisions, like the provision of a phone for a person with a disability. But in general they will experience resources not so much as money (except for their own salary and travel cheques) as in the form of facilities, like hours of home help time, or spaces in a residential or day care unit.

Under a system of care management this changes, whether the care manager is the budget holder or not. In the first place, imagination and flexibility in assessments and care plans will be of limited value if they are circumscribed by a complex and rigid structure of existing budgetary categories. Flexibility of service response means that a much higher proportion of resources will have to be held in flexible form – in essence as money which can be used to purchase a variety of services. Second, the increased involvement of the independent sector means that budgets cannot be tied to direct service provision, but must be available for 'shopping', that is, to buy services from external agencies. Social services departments will already have a fund like this, for example to pay for a specialised residential place not available internally, and it will need to be massively extended. Third, traditional central control of budgets by finance staff will have to be replaced by extensive devolution. Care managers or their service managers need budgets to purchase care packages: not just budgets on paper as part of an internal transfer system, but real budgets to buy what is agreed for their clients.

This in turn puts the spotlight on the way in which such budgets can be provided. For example, care management can be treated as something of an appendage to mainstream activity, a bit of a side show, operating on the equivalent of a petty cash basis. Or it can be treated as important but separate from other servicing systems, with an earmarked ('ring-fenced') budget. Both of these are feasible if the social services department moves just a little way into care management, perhaps for the community care of clients who are mentally ill or have disabilities or learning difficulties. However it is hard to see why, if care management delivers the outcomes expected of it, any agency should want to retain the cumbersome framework where part of a client load is serviced through one system and the remainder through another. Care management could then become the mainstream system, funded by way of total budgetary devolution to front line localities.

Care management in context

The further the debate moves into budgetary matters, the clearer it becomes that these are set to force their attention onto social workers and enter the scene as new demands on time and requirements for new knowledge and skills. In contrast, part of the last chapter sought to establish that care management is not a novelty, but something consistent with established forms of practice, in this instance with the role of key worker. Between these extremes of new departure and old practice there are ways in which care management encourages attention to particular aspects of traditional professional practice, noticeably in the vital areas of assessment and the organisation of service delivery.

Assessment has always been at the heart of good social work, both because the accuracy of its content determines the relevance of subsequent interventions, and because the process brings worker and client together and sets the course for their continuing relationship. In some circumstances the client gains considerably from a thorough, sensitive and systematic assessment, which makes a direct contribution to achieving improvements or awareness of whatever problems are identified. In other circumstances an assessment can be restrictive and unhelpful because it is impossible for the worker (often also the client) to remain unaware of service potential. As we have already asked, what is the point of working comprehensively through a client's needs, if these are not going to be met?

Care management does not have the answer, but it does stress the importance of not trying to fit people to resources they do not want or to which they are not suited. Like any other system it depends in the last resort on resources being available, and lack of resources will demoralise client and worker alike. In two ways, however, care management seeks to emphasise the value of a full assessment, though both are likely to provoke scathing rejoinders from some professional workers. One is contained in the view that clients may not have a right to service, but do have a right to be assessed. This extends to social work the principle which has always applied to welfare benefits – that you may not qualify for any benefit, but you have a right to have your eligibility fully calculated. The other emerges from the suggestion that the absolute rigidity of resource decisions based wholly on public funding can be given more flexibility if scope exists to raise resources elsewhere, such as through fund raising by the client's family and friends.

The organisation of intervention, including possible resource gathering, stresses the roles of co-ordinator and enabler. Both, as discussed, have a firm base in traditional practice, and there is little doubt that care management contains important elements of the role of the key worker and the community worker, especially the former. However the care manager's position is significantly stronger. As we indicated earlier, the key worker seeks to co-ordinate, but may function from a weak position, as, for example, when trying to hold together activity (or overcome inactivity) in a service team which contains staff in higher status or hierarchically senior posts. The care manager may be placed in the same situation, for example when trying to co-ordinate the work of medical consultants, but is potentially strengthened by control of the resource strings and by the fact of the care package having been negotiated and contracted. In the last resort the care manager, as purchaser of services, may be able to reject a service, or move a service provision away from an unsatisfactory provider, which is something no key worker can do.

The independent sector

Implicit in the above paragraphs is the notion of the care manager as the organiser of service provision, rather than the direct provider. At this point we will consider more closely one aspect of the organisational task – working with the independent sector.

Britain has passed through nearly half a century in which public responsibility for personal social services has been established, with such major landmarks as the formation of Children's Departments in 1948 and Social Services Departments in 1971. The steady trend has not only been towards public provision, but to the pivotal role of the local authority. Throughout this period there has been a model of a social services worker whose task is to enable service rather than provide it directly. This concept will be familiar to community workers, who emphasise the key role of local people in deciding about and implementing measures to improve their circumstances; or community organisers, who see their task as co-ordinating diverse activities to help them achieve a sense of coherence; or group workers seeking to promote self-help and mutual aid within client groups. A more explicitly generic extension of the enabling function in social work is found in the Barclay Report, especially Hadley's minority statement (Barclay, 1982), in the job description of the community social worker, and in practice in communities like Normanton (Hadley and McGrath, 1980) where a patch system operates.

For the 1990s we can expect that this approach will be

much extended, moving beyond the idea that individual social workers and others should 'enable' as well as 'do', to the view of agencies as enablers. In the words of *Caring for People* (Department of Health, 1989, para.1.11), a key objective for service delivery will be 'to promote the development of a flourishing independent sector alongside good quality public services'. To achieve this it will be the responsibility of local authorities 'to make maximum possible use of private and voluntary providers, and so increase the available range of options and widen consumer choice'.

The independent sector is made up of three sorts of organisation – voluntary group, non-profit agency and private company – along with assorted individuals or groups involved in such activities as advocacy, campaigning and development trials. If in any area these bodies do not exist or are too small to make an impact, then the local authority is expected to take action to help create or improve what the government calls a 'mixed economy of care'. There are various ways an independent sector can be promoted, including invitations to groups to tender for specific service provisions, encouraging local authority staff to make bids to take over, on a private basis, functions currently handled by the authority, or offering appropriate training.

Local authorities are not required to contract out their services unless the arrangement is cost effective (that is, it would cost less if handled privately than it would if provided directly by the local authority), but they will have to incur expenditure and workload regardless of where the cost advantages lie. They have to help the independent sector get into the position where it can make and implement competitive bids, and at the same time retain a capacity for direct provision in case the independent sector fails.

The powers to negotiate a care package, monitor the work of service providers and, as a last resort, to change provider, derive from the classic relationship between wealth and power, paying the piper and calling the tune. In practice they are powers which may formally rest with the service manager, that is, the care manager's own line manager, but their location at the service front line is a massive empowerment of social workers and their immediate colleagues . . . as long as an adequate budget is available.

Devolution and consumerism

Devolution and consumerism are linked in this context because they share a common motivation, which is to place decision making more firmly at the interface of client and worker. The argument for devolution in care management is about the authority, most critically the extent of control over resources (discussed above), which is devolved down the hierarchy to the service manager and then on to the care manager. The consumerist issue is then about the extent to which the client, along with carer or advocate, can share in the exercise of this authority.

Devolution

In traditional social work practice there is a complex mix of devolved and centralised authority. The nature of social work, based on transactions between client and worker, and dealing so often with urgent situations, requires considerable discretion to reside with the social worker or immediate supervisor. This professional discretion is inevitable and generally accepted as such. However, many proposed interventions with or on behalf of clients have resource implications, and increasingly front line staff are expected to refer up the hierarchy for approval of potentially costly actions. This is more obvious, and more necessary, where substantial cost is involved, as when bringing a young person into residential care, possibly for many years. It is likely to be more flexibly handled where much smaller costs occur. The whole system is overlaid by the notion of accountability, which is a mixture of compulsory procedures for seeking approval for actions and the expectation that devolved authority or professional discretion will be exercised responsibly.

The ideas behind care management do not so much conflict with these traditional approaches, as imply two faults which need correcting. One concerns the perceived sloppiness of current decision-making processes where there are costs, because they do not permit tight financial bookkeeping. The solution to this weakness is to ensure that all care packages are fully costed before any decision is taken on implementation. The second relates to the complex and confused way that cost-related decisions are spread throughout the agency hierarchy, with no-one having an up-to-date overview. Under one model of care management this problem can be overcome. Senior agency managers set budget ceilings for given services in a geographical area over a specified period, and the allocation of those funds is then devolved to the service or care manager. In practice such devolution may well be closely linked with the sub-office (for example, area centre) structure of the agency.

If the theory of devolution sounds simple, the practice will be much harder. Budgetary devolution is a sensitive and controversial matter, not least because a move to devolve always arouses counter-pressures to reassert centralisation, and vice versa. Control of resources is a well established and recognised power base, and those who favour centralised control are likely to have a strong conviction that devolution, far from being a route to orderly and effective book keeping, is a recipe for budgetary chaos.

Consumerism

The same concerns about the impact of spreading responsibility influence views about the role of consumers. *Caring for People* advocates giving consumers information and some choice, and encourages the use of advocates, but does not mention such notions as 'empowerment'. The origins of consumerist approaches are more basic, and the arguments are attractive to many front line staff. Several ways to achieving greater consumer involvement are possible within the care management framework. They include:

1. giving the client full and detailed information, including access to the 'catalogue' of services available, cost, quality, and so forth;
2. maximising service choices, possibly by considering coupons or vouchers which clients can convert into their chosen service;
3. adding client (or client's representative) views to official records;
4. allowing users' committees to participate in the planning process;
5. promoting and supporting individual voluntarism, including the notion of the client–volunteer; and
6. seeking to appoint helpers to 'fix it' for clients: that is, advocates.

This last point links closely with promoting advocacy, perhaps by sponsoring training and recruitment drives, but crucially through a stated willingness to work with an advocate. To date many agencies have resisted advocates except in relation to people with learning difficulties, but care management offers an opportunity for reconsideration.

A consumer-led input to new forms of community care also permits a more sensitive and realistic appreciation of consumers as a body. There is a long tradition of categorising clients of the personal social services according to the statutory group in which they come for intervention purposes (like the chronically sick and disabled), the type of need they present, the specialism of the worker or team offering service, or the preferred method of intervention. In short, just about every possible category is used except one related to the social, economic and cultural context in which clients carry on their lives.

A closer consumer focus would make the service providers more aware of those features of our society which advantage and disadvantage citizens. In particular, it will be possible to take note of forms of discrimination, on account of gender, race and other characteristics, which are so bound in as causal factors in the emergence of problems, as impediments to effective self-help, and as inhibitors of sensitive client–worker transactions. This can be achieved by several practical routes. One is to consider employing for potential clients the sort of equal opportunities monitoring which a growing number of organisations now use for job applicants, whereby confidential information is gathered and used to check and, if necessary rectify, any discrimination. Another is to use such information about potential clients more rigorously as a basis for the staffing and resource balance of personal social services agencies. An obvious illustration is to match the languages of staff to those of potential clients. Care management is a system for ensuring, on a wider basis, an appropriate match of client needs to service provision.

A rather different approach to consumer circumstances is to reduce (but not abandon) agency use of client categorisation which is based either on in-house convenience or problem labelling, and, where appropriate, to use more pertinent indicators. Hence, alongside categories like 'people with disabilities' or 'elderly mentally infirm' we have groupings like 'below poverty line income' and 'dependent on female carer'. In such cases the presentation of the agency's caseload would have an additional consumer-focused dimension, and more importantly, such categories are used in the process of resource earmarking.

Ultimately, as the list above shows, the most effective measures towards consumerism are linked with the devolution of information, decision making and resources to the consumers themselves.

Summary

In this chapter we have sought to address at a general level some of the overarching themes of care management. In doing this we have highlighted what is new and different in care management for social workers. Themes have included the emphasis on consumer choice, a move towards budgetary devolution and the direct linking of front line decisions to resources. These particular policy initiatives will involve front line social workers in activities which are new to them, such as resource generating, and in areas of decision making which have to date not been their concern. In addressing the criticism that care management, as envisaged, is dominated by budgetary provision we have acknowledged that this may be so but that this is not merely a one-way process. Actions taken by care managers will be controlled by budgetary considerations, but those actions will also influence budgetary considerations. Hence the identification of service providers, the level of assessment and the heightening of consumer awareness will all have an impact on levels of service provision.

We maintain that the practice of care management is central. So far we have made assumptions that care managers will be social workers. This is not necessarily the case, but there are many reasons why they should hold key roles in the care management process, as we outline in Chapter 4. In this chapter we have begun to indicate how care management will have a major impact upon the social work profession. These include the expectation that services can be provided from a number of sources, including the independent sector, voluntary, private and 'not for profit' organisations, and the assumption that social services departments will no longer be the sole provider of services and in some cases may, in fact, be the purchaser of services on behalf of clients or allow clients to purchase for themselves, as true 'consumers'. Before moving to a detailed examination of the tasks involved it is important to analyse how significantly different the philosophy of care management is from the generally accepted values of social work.

3

Building upon Present Practice

Introduction

In the first two chapters we commented upon the shift from
residential care to community care, identifying this, alongside many other developments, as one of the precursors to
care management. In doing so we acknowledged that the
concerns of social workers about care management were
threefold. The first concern, that it is dominated by budgetary and resource matters, has been addressed and will be
returned to at various points in the text. The second, that
although the language has changed there is nothing new in
care management, will be explored in the next two chapters.
There is a counter argument which is that care management
will undermine basic social work values and practices, and
this will also be explored in the next two chapters. The aim
of this chapter is to identify some common strands between
the principles and practices of care management and current
social work practice. In this we will seek to identify whether
care management constitutes a major challenge or change in
direction for social work, or whether it can be seen as part of
a continuum of flexible and developing practice.

Challenge to practice

It has been generally recognised that, at the start of the 1990s, social workers have begun to express real concern about the implementation of care management (Allen, 1990). Is this merely resistance to the challenge which is being offered and if so what is the basis for this resistance? One significant aspect of the recommendations in *Caring for People* (Department of Health, 1989) is that policy makers have shown increasing awareness of the way social workers in the past have invoked the sanctuary of the one-to-one client–worker relationship to resist changes to the way services are provided.

A sequence of legislation (in child care, Child Care Act 1980; mental health, Mental Health Act 1983 and criminal justice, Powers of the Criminal Court Act 1983) has endeavoured to bring about changes in practice, but has largely failed to move social workers either from a traditional attitude about the 'ownership' of clients or from traditional working patterns. History suggests that other policy initiatives similarly have failed to impinge upon the behaviour of social workers. For example, in the personal social services the Seebohm Report (1968) and its thrust towards generic social work was short-lived, and by the mid-1970s there had begun a new move towards specialisation according to client group (Parsloe and Stevenson, 1978). The hotly defended stances in the minority reports to the Barclay Report (1982) and the failure of the majority report to influence either policy or practice reflect the difficulties of bringing about change, even in a climate which questioned the efficacy of social work practice (Rees, 1978; Brewer and Lait, 1980; Sheldon, 1978). Similar defensiveness and resistance can be plotted within the probation service. Innovations in the range of sentences did little to move either probation officers or sentencers from a dependence upon the traditional operation of the probation order as a means of supervising offenders. The Statement of National Objectives and Priorities (SNOP,

1985) demanded that local area probation services respond to its recommendations by identifying services other than casework, and the critique of the treatment model from within the profession is long-standing (Bottoms and McWilliams, 1979). However it is the current policy document, the Green Paper, *Supervision and Punishment in the Community: A framework for action* (Home Office, 1990) on reorganisation of the management structure of the service and, equally importantly, the implications of a Resource Management Information System (1990), which are more likely to achieve the changes that policy makers are demanding.

Likewise, it is in the detailed expectations of organisation for care management that the real challenge to the social work task might come. We will consider these in the next section of the book, but before doing so it is important to consider further the underlying principles and, in the first instance, look at whether in changing the practice there is any fundamental challenge to the values of social work.

Congruence

Having said that there is a challenge implicit in the legislation and policy directives of the 1990s for both the personal social services and the probation service, it is ironic that commentators on care management have also chosen to highlight the congruence between aspects of the innovations and the traditional social work stance. Hence Renshaw comments, 'The most fundamental objectives of case management [*sic*] programmes share the general set of values which lie behind most social services and social work practice' (1988, p. 81). This is a sentiment shared by Beardshaw when she denies any magical qualities of care management and suggests the ingredients are 'simply good practice that has been around for a long time' (1990, p. ii). Much of the language of commentaries on community, consumer choice and empowerment is not merely acceptable but embodies the philosophies that many social workers have espoused over the last two or three decades. Similarly the arguments that initiatives in the new criminal justice legislation are concerned with working with offenders in the community and keeping them out of custody might seem hard to refute. What causes problems is the planned implementation of these concepts in a way that appears intrinsically alien to those working in the statutory social services. At the root of resistance is the intention that such aims should be achieved by a mixed economy of welfare, ending the role of the local authority or the probation service as the major direct service provider.

At one level there would appear to be nothing wrong with such moves. They are congruent with some of the basic tenets of social work, as Cooper points out: 'Even if you think of individualized packages of care drawn from the public, private and voluntary sectors as a market model, it remains a paradox that this view of community care inherits the casework tradition of responding to individual need by listening to the users' understanding of their needs' (Cooper, 1989, p. 187).

It is Beardshaw's seemingly contradictory assertion that, in choosing a particular model of care management, social services will have to accept 'a major shift in social work methods for many staff' which presents the conundrum for social workers. How will there be change and no change? This conundrum is further complicated for those working in the criminal justice system when there is a redefinition of the underlying principles of their work. For the probation service they will no longer be *caring* in the community, they will be *punishing*.

Change

There is no doubt that there will be changes. At the most obvious level, the language has changed. Throughout this text we identify, utilise and try to give some definitions for the terms which are to become the lexicon of social work of the 1990s. This concern with language is not new. In 1984, when the Home Office issued its Statement of National Objectives and Priorities (SNOP) the National Association of Probation Officers were quick to comment that the term 'social work' occurs only once. Similarly Bamford (1990) comments on the infrequency of the term in the Griffiths Report. The question is how significant is the changing terminology and whether the new language will be accompanied by other more radical changes, thus bringing to an end the power of 'the tail of social work to wag the personal social services dog' (Webb and Wistow, 1987, p. 208).

In the case of the probation service already given there would appear to be a significant difference between *caring* and *punishing*, but does it make any difference to the activities of probation officers? If the underlying values are constant, if care management represents 'good practice' and if punishing people in the community keeps them out of penal institutions, then what changes are required? Are they merely changes in the way services are delivered or in the personnel who deliver them? Are they more fundamental? At what level will they occur? Those recommended by Hadley and Young (1990), for example, seem to imply that major organisational change is necessary, as is a preparedness on the part of social workers to 'like it or lump it'. If that is so, then an initial indication is that social workers are 'lumping it', leaving in large numbers and not being replaced by new recruits (NALGO, 1989).

Organisational change is also implicit in the recommendations of Smale and Tuson when they advocate a community social work approach which will go beyond the 'monolithic' organisation (1990, p. 152). This approach seems inherently positive for both individual workers and organisations, presuming they can respond to the change. Perhaps here is the difference: that this change is responsive to innovative practice rather than reactive to management imposition, so local initiatives by individuals and teams in local authority social services and in probation practice can be accepted and broadcast, encouraging and inspiring others.

However the major change anticipated and feared by social workers is the intention in the move towards diversification to remove financial responsibility for welfare from the state, and in doing so to challenge many of the underlying philosophies of the welfare state. The real concerns of front line social workers and probation officers alike are twofold – that their own profession will be undermined and that the people for whom they have a responsibility, the clients, will receive a service which is underfunded and which is provided on principles of profit rather than as a response to need.

These are very real fears, but it is important to acknowledge that a commitment to a welfare state is no longer universally accepted. There is also the possibility that the pressure to reorganise service delivery offers opportunities to meet some of the criticisms of current practice and enhance service quality. It is our intention to explore some of these criticisms in the light of the changes envisaged as a consequence of community care legislation, and to identify some positive ways of taking on the challenge.

A shared set of values

Ever since Towle (1965) attempted to identify social work practice based on common human needs, arguments have raged around what social workers do and the purpose for which they do it. The BASW definition suggests social work is 'directed towards enhancing the personal and social functioning of an individual, family, group or neighbourhood' (1977, p. 19); while Davies (1981) maintains it is about maintenance, and others (for example, Haines, 1975) say it is about change.

Underpinning all these definitions, however, are a set of

values which do appear to be acknowledged by most, if not all, commentators. These include respect for persons, individualisation, self-determination and confidentiality. In identifying similarities in the various lists of values Horne (1987) argues that respect for persons and client self-determination are central to most social work thinking and practice. In the context of care management it is significant that the core concepts of individualisation and self-determination have been presented as being at the heart of the move towards consumer choice and the mixed economy of service provision. Is it cynical to suggest that these values have been highlighted because they have resonance for social workers? Cynicism or not, it is useful to explore the use of these values in the policy initiatives and identify the potential for the future practice of social work.

Individualisation

'Designing packages of services tailored to meet the assessed needs of individuals and their carers' (Department of Health, 1989, para.3.1.3). The suggestion here is that social servicing has always been concerned with individuals and that care management is a means by which individual need can be identified and met through individually designed packages. This is wholly consistent with an early definition of individualisation: 'It is the absolute presupposition, so it is argued, of modern casework that clients are not regarded as fulfilling certain types and paradigms but as presenting a particular problem which needs to be considered against its own particular background' (Plant, 1970, p. 9). In the language of the 1990s we might want to substitute 'set of needs' for 'problem', but other than that the principle appears to hold true.

However it is important to recognise that this principle has been open to criticism over the decades. Two major criticisms are relevant. The first is from the philosophical literature itself which asks how social workers ensure that their practice reflects values, how they maintain an individualised approach when their own actions are mediated through a host of variables. These variables include agency function, the resources available and the range of people with whom social workers need to work both as clients and as service providers (Horne, 1987, p. 73). This critique is particularly pertinent when a value is being espoused in a culture where the underlying motivation for changes in the provision of welfare is the need for cost-effectiveness, 'to secure better value for taxpayers' money by introducing a new funding structure for social care' (Department of Health, 1989, para.1.11). Can the stated aims of care management, individually designed packages of care to meet specific needs and cost-effective measures which will achieve value for taxpayers' money, be reconciled without losing the essence of individualisation?

Let us consider an example. A 60 year old woman suffering from arthritis and the after-effects of a stroke was cared for by her husband for some years. She was wheelchair-bound and had refused rehousing to a bungalow because 'they could cope'. The husband died and there was a re-assessment. To enable her to continue coping would require major alterations to the council house and a large scale input of domiciliary services. The pressure was very much that she should move to some sort of sheltered accommodation and release the council house.

The pressure here was one of expedience as well as economy. There was a pressure on council housing in this area but there were places in the sheltered provision. An individual package of care could be, and ultimately was, provided, but only after some effective advocacy on the part of the woman's son.

The second criticism is that individualisation has contributed to an individual culture which has created an over-dependence upon casework and one-to-one work as a method of intervention. The source of this view is the 'radical critique' of the 1970s, but it has been developed in the

1980s by feminist commentators on the provision of social services. Both of these groups (Corrigan and Leonard, 1978; Wilson, 1980) have suggested that individualisation, where the individual's personal experience is seen to be the valid focus for intervention, can serve to pathologise the individual and inhibit any notion of collective or political action. Much of the policy initiative of the late 1980s has been sympathetic to a definite rejection of concepts of casework. This has been very apparent in the development of thinking within the Home Office about the role of the probation service, and is apparent, at a central level, in considerations about the role of the local authority social worker. This is not to suggest that current policy was influenced either by radical thinking from the left or feminism, of whatever political hue. However the view that individualisation can inhibit collective or political action is not tackled by the changes in practice suggested for care management. Indeed it could be argued that care management runs counter to the some of the principles of community *action* even if it does seek to enhance and extend community *care*.

As long as need is identified only as individual need and met by individualised packages of care, even though this may be provided within the community, a number of consequences will ensue. The first is that the burden of care will be placed within the individual sphere, and this traditionally means that women within the family will be called upon to provide the informal caring or to become the army of volunteers for the supported carers. The evidence for this has been well documented (Finch and Groves, 1983). An argument is made that, if packages of care are properly costed and carers paid, this in some way will relieve the situation for women carers. However the implications of moving into a contractual arrangement, even if it is properly funded, has significant implications for women carers. Payment may have the effect of entrapping women into caring, limiting their career choice rather than freeing them. There is also the suggestion that women care out of a sense of 'duty' and that they would be resistant to payment for this duty, as it would merely add to their sense of guilt.

Second, if the response to need is only at an individual level, there will be no acknowledgement of the extent of need, nor will there be any evaluation of the effectiveness of meeting it, other than at the individual care package level. This is significant because often the individual circumstances of need can be the result of policy decisions or of norms and expectations within our society. Much of the critique of service delivery which identifies discriminatory practice on the basis of class, gender and race demonstrates that individual circumstances can arise out of lack of appropriate service delivery in a variety of spheres. Hence the high proportion of women and black people who are recipients of the mental health services, and the higher incidence of some diseases in certain classes, relate both to their individual experiences within society and to the response which they receive from those who provide the services.

It is not appropriate, nor is it cost effective to meet need only at the level of the individual and the expedient. What is required is a collation of information to identify the root cause and action which involves change at a wider policy level. For example, Ungerson argues that, rather than cash support for individual carers, 'what is needed is high quality and easily available day care *services* combined with equally high quality forms of flexible residential care, including permanent sheltered housing for protected independent living and regular respite care for those normally cared for informally' (1987, p. 155). This would provide an ideal package of care which would demand the organising of services at a truly community level rather than a series of responses at the individual level.

The appeal of individual packages of care or the individually tailored sentence within the community is persuasive, and matching resources to individual need might be appropriate, but it is important that the activity of the social worker does not merely end in the provision of the individual package. If this were to happen then care management might merely have similar outcomes to individual casework, the individual being perceived as the problem and the package of care set up to deal with that problem. The opportunity that care management offers is the identification of patterns of need related to circumstances of groups of clients based on a variety of common denominators, which may include social class, race or gender as well as definitions of the illness or disability. To do this requires systems for collating information and aggregating data to be designed at the local level as well as at the regional and county level; however, it will also require a change of attitude on behalf of social workers.

Self-determination and consumer choice

'Give people a greater individual say in how they live their lives and the services they need to help them do so.' (*Caring for People*, Department of Health, 1989, para.1.8). There is little in the concept of consumer choice with which social workers will disagree. Apart from connotations of individualisation, it also has embedded in it the notion of self-determination, a long standing principle in social work (Biestek, 1961; Plant, 1970). Despite its primacy of place in the canon of social work literature, this concept is open to widely differing interpretations. While care management, by devolving budgets and diversifying services, seeks to widen the possibilities of providing care within the community and to give consumers some influence over that provision, it too is open to these criticisms of self-determination.

In the first instance it is acknowledged that anyone's capacity for self-determination is limited by the needs of others to be equally self-determining. Within community care the involvement of informal carers is an example of the dilemma created. The ability of the individual to lead some form of independent life in the community is dependant upon levels of service which so often can only be provided by those who have emotional ties to them. The reality is that for a number of reasons – socialisation, guilt, social pressure or pure altruism – the majority of informal caring in this country is taken on by women. The assumption that a female member of a family will at least give serious consideration to providing unpaid and informal care is the basis on which many social workers have proceeded over the years.

While not openly acknowledging the gendered sex role stereotypes in the assumptions about caring, the policy of informal caring recognises the reality 'that most care is provided by family, friends and neighbours. The majority of carers take on these responsibilities willingly, but the Government recognises that many need help to be able to manage what can become a heavy burden' (Department of Health, 1989, para.2.3).

Whatever the sex of the carer the context of informal caring is one which is riddled with conflicting and competing needs. These are realities for the carer and for the individual consumers who, in desiring their own independence, are also acutely aware of the demands that they may have to make and the 'burden' they may become. What this requires from social workers, according to Pitkeathley (1990), is a change in the relationship between professional and carer which not only acknowledges the needs of carers in their own right but also recognises the special role that they fulfil which is separate and different from the professional carer.

Take another example. An elderly couple living in a warden controlled flat have to cope with the husband's need for heart surgery. Post operation, he is due to be moved to a convalescent home but he insists that, as his wife is a qualified SRN, she is capable of looking after him. While she agrees to this she identifies that she can carry out the technical skills but that the negotiations over diet and behaviour are fraught because of the nature of the interpersonal relationship: 'He is not just Mr. S. in bed 3, he is *my* John and I need him to get well.'

There is potential in care management to afford carers a different status. Additionally, while consumerism suggests that individuals, whether frail elderly or adults with learning difficulties, should have the right to choose, Pitkeathley (1990) rightly argues that carers also ought to have the right to choose. However, for a number of reasons, many carers feel that they have little choice. 'Ring-fenced' funding for carers might go part way to redressing some of the imbalances in their position, but there are also some basic issues about the negotiating position of carers which have significant connotations for care management and the social work task. The assessment process will be critical in ensuring that the needs of carers are addressed and that there are not automatic assumptions made by the social worker, or the person in need of care, about the resources, human and otherwise, at the disposal of those being assessed.

The second set of criticisms is to do with the inference that individuals, be they consumers or carers, are able to make choices and that the individual knows what s/he wants (or in this case needs) and that s/he is able to demand it if it is not available. Users of the social services tend to represent groups who have not been socialised into asserting their needs, or have been told consistently that they have no status or right to demand. Among these are the lower socio-economic groups and women from all classes. There are also a number of groups who have remained outside provision because their needs have traditionally been ignored or misinterpreted by statutory social workers, mainly groups within the ethnic minority communities (Dominelli, 1988; Ely and Denny, 1987).

The implication of this for care management is that to ensure effective community care provision social workers need to work with clients to enable them to express their needs. At the same time full information on the possible range of services has to be given, even where these might not be readily available, and to provide or acquire them might involve the social worker in a great deal of effort. This may seem to require a different set of skills for social workers, but they are not totally new. Priestley *et al.* (1978) addressed the need to provide clients with appropriate social skills. What is perhaps more challenging is the requirement in cases where, for whatever reason, clients or carers are not able to express their needs, that the social worker will act as an advocate, demanding a quality of service from the very agency that employs them.

Thus it becomes clear that, while there are some resonances between the values of social work and the principles of care management in community care, there are also some unresolved issues which need to be addressed. We acknowledged at the beginning of this chapter that social work had resisted many challenges to its traditional methodologies. When faced with the opportunity to move away from one-to-one working and link in a more integrated way with individuals, families and communities, social workers have tended to hold firm to the individual interpersonal relationship, even if they no longer accept the theories of Freud as a basis for this relationship. The implication of this is that social workers are at risk of continuing to make assessments which identify individuals' needs as involving support and counselling rather than a whole package of practical assistance.

This tenacity in remaining firmly in the mould of the caseworker will not necessarily achieve that positive aim of community care policy which is to facilitate the individual living independently in the community for as long as possible. Asking people how they feel does not ensure that they are being properly fed or are assisted into their beds at night. Can the person survive physically despite their emotional turmoil? Counselling or support may be identified as a critical component of the care that is needed, but this need not necessarily be provided by the statutory social worker, who could instead arrange for specialist counselling agencies or specially recruited and trained volunteers to be 'contracted in'.

The significance of this set of issues is that, while care management has the potential to draw upon and be even more effective in ensuring that some basic values are adhered to, much of this potential is dependent upon the activities of individual workers who will prepare the assessment and deliver the packages of care. Within the process of care management there are specific points at which there are opportunities to change practice and we will expand on these in the next chapter.

Community care: equality of opportunity?

Before moving on, however, there is one further set of issues to be considered in a discussion about building upon present practice. Over the last ten years there have been criticisms about discriminatory aspects of social work practice, especially on the basis of race and gender (Brook and Davis, 1985; ADSS/CRE, 1989). In making specific reference to the needs of people from ethnic minorities, *Caring for People* (1989, para.2.9) indicates that the government is at least aware of some of these criticisms and seeks to address them. It is important therefore to examine the potential for change within the legislation and policy initiatives and how they relate to equality of opportunity in social work. To do this we need to clarify some concepts.

The first is that of equal access. There are competing principles within the community care policies themselves. On the one hand it is made clear that it is not the intention of community care that anyone and everyone needing some form of care in the community should be referred to social services departments. It is acknowledged that some individuals have the capacity for problem solving and negotiating their own support systems. On the other hand the policy for all those over 75 years does embody a universal right to assessment, even if it does not ensure a universal right to services.

Although the widening of the net, the attempt to provide universal access to services, might be seen to have beneficial consequences and to embody the best principles of equal opportunities, it is important to recognise that there are also some drawbacks. The reality is that, even though individuals are said to be given more self-determination within the proposed changes, the concept of 'clientism' within social service provision, when becoming a client involves becoming the object of a whole series of assumptions and subject to all sorts of investigation, can in itself amount to discriminatory practice. While consumers might have more choice within care management, becoming a user of social services does involve the giving up of citizenship rights and imposes certain restrictions (Gregory, 1987). In many ways some of the existing discriminatory practices have led to the inappropriate inclusion of certain groups in social service provision, for example the over-representation of black children in residential care. Equality of opportunity in community care is therefore not just a matter of getting people into the system; it also involves balance, safeguarding against unfair discrimination to ensure access is possible for those who might be in need of the services, so that no one in need goes without a service, but no one is brought into the welfare net inappropriately.

Much of this concerns individual worker activity in the process of care management, but there are some wider aspects which are also relevant and relate to the second concept, that of equal treatment. Section 71 of the 1976 Race Relations Act confers on local authorities particular duties to ensure that they eliminate unlawful racial discrimination and promote equality of opportunity and good relations between persons of different racial groups. In 1989, a report by the Commission for Racial Equality (CRE) and the Association of Directors of Social Services revealed that, despite the legislation, social service departments had made little progress with their policies to do with race. Many had equal opportunities policies, but few had any specific strategy either to eliminate racist practice or to ensure that their services were ethnically sensitive and appropriate to the needs of minority groups within their area. The CRE further point out that, as a function of local authority service provision, community care is also covered by the Race Relations Act 1976. In stating that 'where there is equal need there has to be equal treatment' (1990b) they go on to reiterate the point – made by so many other commentators on local authority service provision – that there is not adequate provision for members of ethnic minority communities. Equal treatment is not just to do with treating everyone the same, assuming that services constructed according to white norms will meet the needs of black and ethnic minority people. As Forbes (1989) points out, equality of treatment does not guarantee equality of opportunity, this depends on having appropriate responses to identified need, thereby giving black and ethnic minority people equal rights to have their needs met.

This provision does not only depend on individual worker activity, but requires policy initiative and guidance at an organisational level. Within the recommendations for diversification of services comes a real possibility for consultation about needs and co-operating with representatives of communities to ensure that needs are identified and appropriate provision is made so that local authorities ensure non-discriminatory provision and practice. For example, access to services will be much more effective if community groups, at the level of the Race Equality Councils and voluntary organisations, can be supported both to disseminate information and be service providers. This is not to marginalise but to ensure that the service delivery is communicable and responsive to the cultural norms of different racial groups. If this is accompanied by devolution of budgets to the individual clients then this will allow them effective choice and not just a choice between inappropriate services.

Such an approach can increase the opportunity for services to become more client-centred. For women, for example, the Birmingham Women and Social Work Group's analysis of the dilemma of feminist practice within state welfare highlighted that even workers committed to anti-discriminatory practice had to work within the limitations of agency policy and practice (Brook and Davis, 1985). One way forward is to acknowledge that 'Alternative resources set up by women and for women are invaluable, not only because we can refer our clients to them for specific types of help and support, but also because they serve as models for the future developments of state services' (1985, p. 121). This hope of the 1980s was never realised, but the policy changes of the 1990s might enable women to set up resources in the community which will become a provision in their own right rather than a blueprint for services provided by the state.

Properly resourced and funded, the potential for women centred support as a community care provision is enormous. This is particularly relevant when we consider that the majority of the ageing population are women and that women constitute a greater proportion of the users of the mental health services. The example of Women's Aid and Rape Crisis demonstrates that services run by women for women have been extremely effective in areas where the state has failed to make an appropriate provision. It can be argued that in many areas of provision statutory services have failed to recognise the particular needs of women (Hanmer and Statham, 1988) and that care management in community care provides an opportunity to redress this.

Thus it can be seen that the implementation of care management in community care could offer the opportunity to redress some of the weaknesses in current social work practice, particularly in relation to discriminatory practice. It is not being argued that care management sets out to address issues of equal opportunities in the service delivery of social work agencies, but that the move away from individualised intervention and a treatment model, coupled with the diversification of service provision, offers opportunities to build on good practice.

In many ways diversification of services and budgetary devolution could mean that the example set by voluntary groups such as MIND, the Independent Living Foundation and the National Schizophrenia Fellowship, who have acted as advocates and have set excellent examples of involving users in the provision of service, can be expanded upon. However it is also important to heed the message from such groups, that for this approach to be effective it needs, like all other forms of formal service provision, to be properly funded and resourced and afforded equal status.

Summary

In this chapter we have tried to take the overview of care management in community care a stage further. By addressing the very real concerns that social workers have about the implementation of care management we have suggested that, within limits, there are opportunities to build upon basic social work values, especially those of individualisation and client self-determination. While some of the language might be new, there is some congruence between the aims of traditional social work and those of care management. The argument is that within care management there may also be opportunities to improve social work practice and to address some of the criticisms made on the basis of unfair discrimination. This will contribute to effective implementation of equal opportunities policies. In recognising that the potential exists within care management we acknowledge that there are certain inhibitors. The first is resources. The second is the activity and attitudes of individual workers in the care management process. The next chapter gives a detailed analysis of this process and highlights opportunities for workers to implement best practice. It may be that if best practice identifies the full extent of need then there could be the possibility within budgetary devolution for creative and innovative ways to use the resources.

4

Care Management: Process and Outcomes

Introduction

Social work has always had an element of care organising and enabling alongside direct work with clients. The concept of care management takes the process still further: enabling is mediated through the management of care packages. At the same time care management is not restricted to qualified social workers. Others, such as home care organisers, may be appropriate persons to be care managers, depending on who are the clients. This combination of distancing social workers to some extent from direct work with clients and allowing others to take on the care manager role is one of the bases for assertions that traditional social work skills will be devalued.

We have examined how, properly approached, care management can build upon existing values, but we also need to consider the skills required. New skills are being demanded in care management which, if they had to be embodied in a single person, would dilute and swamp a social work curriculum which is already overloaded. Some of the new tasks, in budgets and fund raising, for example, go beyond demanding new skills: they pose a need for a different kind of person. Social work values have always placed considerable emphasis on the personalities of social workers, justifying such an approach by the argument that working with people, especially people facing stressful intimate difficulties in their lives, demands particular personal aptitudes. What are the chances that the personality which makes a good social worker will also make a good accountant?

The challenge comes also from moves to detach social workers to an extent from direct client work, or to bring other helpers and service providers into the relationship. To someone who views social work as a close and exclusive relationship between therapist (or counsellor) and client this is more than a challenge: it is the demolition of a core value. Yet to others, and this probably makes up the majority of social workers in Britain, the challenge is neither new nor threatening. Those who work in multi-disciplinary teams will be accustomed to sharing client contact with other staff. Many more will routinely relate to clients in collaboration with less qualified colleagues, such as home carers and volunteers. Others will feel familiar with the gregariousness and unpredictability of client relationships in groups or through community activities. If there is a threat in this challenge, it comes perhaps from the possibility that the care manager will be pulled back out of client contact altogether, forced to develop an 'arm's length' relationship, dependent on the behaviour of those less qualified staff who come between care manager and client.

The implications for social workers of these apparent changes are reflected in the more prescriptive statements which relate specifically to the function of providing care management in community care. Such prescriptions had their origins in the Barclay Report (1982) with the identification of social care planning and counselling as distinct activities. There the Pinker and Hadley debate served to illustrate the distinctions, even if they could not agree on who was going to carry out which functions. However with less dissent the Griffiths Report (1988) became more focused and, as Bamford observes, the scant references to social workers in that report either imply the training of social workers into a more managerial role or mean 'that the new role envisaged in designing, organising and purchasing services is so fundamentally different from that currently performed that a wholly different approach is required to which social work has a contribution to make' (Bamford, 1990, p. 159).

We have no analysis of the care management process which offers guidance either on the changes of practice which might constitute this 'wholly different approach' or on the management of these practices.There are a number of documents from the Department of Health on policy guidance (1990), purchase of services (1991a) and assessment (1991b), but none of them address in detail the basic question of what social workers will be required to do. Although the legislation is in place, the practice models on which it draws are diverse. In America, where many of the early care management schemes emerged, the model is built around the specialist care manager, whatever the professional background. The models for operating care management systems in Britain vary both in the way that the service is delivered and in the personnel involved. The Kent experiment, for instance, was run as a research project where the 'community care workers assessed need, supported and advised clients and carers and undertook brokerage and advocacy' (Challis and Davies, 1989, p. 57). At the outset the expectation of smaller caseloads and different ways of working with a client group identified by specific criteria were acknowledged. Other schemes have been more evolutionary. Based in local area centres they have involved non-specialist care managers working on individual programme planning for as many cases as possible (Renshaw, 1988).

This lack of a consistent operational model means that, although there is policy guidance, there are no frameworks, guidelines and systems for the management of the evolving roles and tasks for the individual worker. This is a common phenomenon in British social work, that new practices come about by innovative thinking in methods of intervention or are imposed by major policy changes. Social workers, chameleon like, adapt to these circumstances and only at a later stage realise that their workloads have changed in size or composition and that this has implications for their ability to perform the task. Hence the BASW (1977) analysis of the social work task came some time after the Seebohm reorganisation, and the more recent NALGO study (1989) was precipitated by a crisis of morale and staffing. The need to develop a workload system in tandem with the developments in care management will be outlined in Chapter 7. Before we are able to do this effectively we need to identify the tasks that have to be performed and the skills necessary to perform them. A systematic look at this will leads us to consider who will perform the tasks and the implications of this for those currently employed in various front line social work roles.

What has to be done?

The designing and organising of services is the essence of care management. This has been broken down into five functions in *Caring for People* (1989). These five functions are parallel to the five functions identified by Challis and Davies (1989). (See Table 4.1.)

Table 4.1 *Comparison of the components of care management*

Caring for People (1989, sect.3.3.4, p. 21)	*Challis and Davies (1989, p. 39)*
Identification of people in need	Case finding
Assessment of care needs	Assessment
Planning and securing the delivery of care needs	Case planning and service arrangement
Monitoring the quality of care provided	Monitoring and review
Review of client needs	Closure

The rest of this chapter attempts to clarify the tasks identified as constituting the process of care management. In this clarification it is important to consider the possible ways of organising the various tasks. Does the care manager have to perform all the tasks in the care management process? Is each component task an individual function or an agency function? Is it necessary for every task to be performed by a front line qualified social worker?

Identification of people in need

The alternative title of 'case finding' reflects some of the anomalies in this process. Workloads of social workers have increased and vacancies within the profession have increased, so that there seems to be no shortage of cases or people in need (NALGO, 1989). However, overloaded social services departments do not necessarily mean that all need is being met; it may mean they are under resourced or inefficiently managed.

The implication of a case finding system is that all people in need of a service will be identified, or asked to identify themselves. They will be assessed as to whether they are able, or would wish, to benefit from community care and then become part of the care management process. *Caring for People* and the subsequent legislation appear to limit eligibility by focusing on particular client groups or even individuals within client groups in particular situations, such as long-term hospital care. However the specific provision for the assessment of all those over 75 years of age also widens the potential for a universal eligibility.

This will present a paradox for workers in the social services who have to some extent been searching to create ceilings on workloads and to prioritise the demands which have been made upon agencies. Having spent time attempting to control their workloads they are being asked to respond to all demands. The varied referral systems which agencies have adopted, including intake teams, which do some form of sifting before allocating on for longer-term social work intervention, or open door duty office systems which make instant initial assessments and refer on for further assessment may no longer be appropriate. Since the Seebohm Report (1968) the philosophy has been primarily to offer a service to those who find their way to the agency reception desk, rather than involving the department in a publicity campaign to attract take-up of services. However the Chronically Sick and Disabled Persons Act 1970 did include a requirement to set up a register of those with potential needs. In the Barclay Report (1982) it was further suggested that organising social services on the basis of smaller geographical units would enable the needs of the community to be identified. The suggestion is that, with early identification of needs and the provision of appropriate levels of service within the community, crises which can make more demands of social services resources, both human and residential, can be averted (Hadley and McGrath, 1984).

The proposals embedded in the National Health Service and Community Care Act 1990 add further dimensions to the process of meeting need. In addition to the current practice of individuals presenting themselves at the agency, there are five further aspects of the identification of need:

1. the use of demographic information to try and predict the levels of need within a prescribed geographical area;
2. the early identification of unmet need or even unacknowledged need;
3. the provision of responsive screening services for particular groups;
4. consultation with community and consumer groups to assist the identification of need;
5. registering of those with needs or at risk.

These categories highlight some real dilemmas for social services departments, but they also raise fundamental questions about where the responsibility lies for identifying the needs and the skills required. Is it an individual social work task to become a 'needs detective' or does the responsibility remain at agency level? The reality is that both systems have to operate in order to identify people in need.

When considering demographic predictions the production of area community care plans must draw upon basic information which can be provided by research and information sections of the agency. Geographical descriptions, age, class and ethnic origin of current referrals are not enough by themselves. Critics of Barclay (for example, Allan, 1983) have implied that a real problem with basing planning decisions on current caseloads is that those who present themselves to agencies are those who have no means of informal caring support or whose informal support mechanisms have broken down for a variety of reasons. A further limitation relates to those individuals or groups who are unacceptable to communities because of their behaviour or the risk involved. This suggests that if existing referral patterns are used as predictive factors they will not reflect the true extent of the need. There needs to be a process of identifying the needs of potential users, and to consider the views of those who want help but do not like what is on offer. Social workers' and volunteers' knowledge of areas and networks will have to be part of information which is considered alongside demographic data and information from community groups and voluntary organisations. Social workers themselves become key informants for the data collection process, and the way that the information is made available is critical. Involvement in long discussion meetings, pooling knowledge and information may be counter-productive, but information technology can provide valuable aids to information gathering, storage and retrieval, as we identify later in this book.

Current information gathering processes of the statutory services have been criticised because some groups, particularly those from ethnic minorities, have not had access to appropriate levels of service (Ely and Denny, 1987; Dominelli, 1988). The opening up of services to such groups is important in terms of early preventative work, but the process of accessing illustrates some further complexities in identifying need. Publicising services by leafleting, even if these leaflets are multi-lingual and placed in advice centres where appropriate languages are spoken, may well not be enough. Work will also need to be done with representatives of local communities and consumer groups to ensure that the services are appropriately presented. As the Commission for Racial Equality has emphasised (1990), this work is equally important in areas where there are relatively few members of ethnic minority communities.

For social services departments the issue here is whether such work needs to be done by a specialist team which has responsibility for identifying needs and involves social work skills or whether such marketing techniques will be taken on at management level. For example, making services accessible to members of black and ethnic minority communities involves a personal commitment of white social workers who need to undertake training to ensure that their practice is non-discriminatory (Dominelli, 1988). Ethnically sensitive service delivery at any point in the process involves appropriate policies, properly resourced and mediated by individuals, whether they are social workers or not, who work in non-discriminatory ways.

A critical aspect of both referring clients and identifying needs, whatever the background of the potential user, is to have full information about the agency's policy. *Caring for People* specifies that the means of referral be widely known, as should the criteria for eligibility for assessment (Department of Health, 1989, para.3.2.9). Such criteria have to be established for the information of both service users and consumers, and for the workers involved in the system.

Finally, as with all referral processes, it is necessary to acquire a certain amount of information and become involved with the individual before even initial service decisions can be made. For social workers there is also the sense in which, even if these decisions are made by working to a checklist, they feel a commitment to saying 'no' in the most caring way possible. A major implication of appropriate intervention at this stage is that the individual will feel able to return to the agency if circumstances change, or will be receptive to future intervention by a representative of the agency should this be necessary.

Assessment of care needs

The process of assessment has always been a vital task in social work (Sainsbury, 1970; Curnock and Hardiker, 1979). It is the means by which decisions are made about the level of service involvement and the nature of that involvement. It is within the assessment process, therefore, that the blueprint is established both for the quantity and quality of the service delivery. Consequently in all social work the assessment process has been pivotal. In care management the issues are even more complex, not least because in this context assessment is 'concerned not only with the *needs* of elderly person but also their *strengths* and the identification of obstacles to achieving change' (Challis and Davies, 1989, p. 44).

This widening of the assessment task to something more than the identification of need will be an essential element of care management in community care for all client groups. A corollary to this is that the process of identifying need and matching it to resources will contribute to more effective assessments, assuming that available resources will be more wide-ranging than those provided solely by social services departments.

For example, the assessment process has always required the involvement of a variety of sources of information (Curnock and Hardiker, 1979; Coulshed, 1988). However, the introduction of community care has led to greater expectations about the consultative nature of the task to be performed (Department of Health, 1989; 1990), thus reflecting Renshaw's (1988) finding that all projects that she studied used a multi-disciplinary or multi-agency approach at some point in the assessment. An appropriate assessment in the context of community care, therefore, has to ensure that the views and the desires of the consumer are identified, and in doing this it has to acknowledge that the very definition of 'consumer' is open to discussion. The views of clients and informal carers as consumers are significant, as are the judgements of other professionals. The ensuing assessment is then the basis for service planning, which in community care can be provided from a number of sources. Hence the views of the providers of these resources become a necessary part of the assessment. The assessment itself becomes a significant part of quality assurance, in that it tries to identify the levels and outcomes of service provision against which the work of other agencies may be measured. It in fact becomes part of a contractual agreement with both the consumer and the service providers.

The significance of this is twofold. First, the recommendations for assessment in care management (Department of Health, 1989; 1990) are prescriptive in identifying the people who may be involved in the assessment process (1989, para.3.2.5), but also limit the methods by which the information may be gathered (1989, para.3.2.11), that is the process of doing the assessment. Such administrative policy guidelines for tasks which are deemed 'social work tasks' are not unique. In recent years the Home Office has issued guidelines for the production of the social inquiry report (Home Office, 1986) and the guidelines for assessment of situations involving children under the new Children Act (Department of Health, 1988) indicate that there is increased central control over the actual practice of social work, despite a supposed commitment to devolution of responsibility. Second, the assessment has to be detailed in its identification of needs, exploring what should be offered and the expected outcomes. It has to be informative, analytic and prescriptive. This is particularly important if the person who carries out the assessment is not going to be the care manager.

What constitutes an assessment?

Practice guides will have to include a consideration of both the changing focus of assessment, and the tasks that will have to be performed (see Table 4.2).

Table 4.2 *The tasks involved in assessment*

Focus	Task
Enable the individual to live at home	Identify needs
	Balancing of risks and needs
Multi-problem analysis	Bring to the assessment the perspectives of all the relevant agencies
Take the wishes of the individual consumer into account	Enable communication
	Facilitate advocacy
	Balance the needs of the carer

While the terminology may be new, a detailed look at the tasks involved shows that they are already part of the assessment task which most social workers undertake as part of their daily activities, whether they be part of an intake team, a court probation officer or investigating a child abuse case. Vickery's analysis of the use of an integrated approach to social work (1976) has given us the skills for identifying client systems and those that are involved with them. A first stage would therefore be to interview client and immediate significant others – referral agent and informal carer where they were not the referrer. The purpose of this first stage would be to identify obvious and apparent need and to locate others whose views would have to be sought for the assessment. The process of gathering information can then take a variety of forms. *Caring for People* dismisses costly case conferences, but advocates quick and informal methods (Department of Health, 1989, para.3.2.11) without specifying what these might be. Telephone conversations are perhaps the quickest and most informal, but they are open to all sorts of misinterpretations and later withdrawals of commitment. A system of forms or assessment schedules would ensure that information was documented and could be kept on file for future use, but failure to complete forms is a common problem. An advantage of a form filling exercise is that, once the list of contributors to an assessment is identified, the task of sending out forms can be devolved to a clerical worker and need not demand too much professional social work time. Eventually such processes can be undertaken by the use of electronic mail and other information technology resources.

However the gathering of information is not the end of the process. Coulshed has highlighted the fact that an assessment is 'a perceptual/analytic process of selecting categorising, organising and synthesising data: it is both a process and a product of our understanding' (1988, p. 13). While it is apparent that analysis, categorising and synthesising data demands a body of knowledge, it is vital that this knowledge is based on experience and skills which are acquired from training and practice. Steinberg and Carter (1983) argue that the most important assessment tool is the well qualified worker who brings to the process skills to do with interviewing techniques. These techniques are informed both by training and by the ability to understand the perceptions and experiences of the participants in the process. This is particularly significant when handling the tensions between carers and those cared for, and in assessing the coping abilities of individuals when information is required about more than their physical state. What needs to be addressed is the feelings, the attitudes and the reactions as well as the basic factual information. Qualified workers can individualise standardised information gathering schedules, and use this to direct the further information they require and the range of people from whom the information is collected. In this way they can co-ordinate the process of the assessment.

There are other factors which may influence the process of assessment in community care. The assessment of those over 75 years old, for example, will have to be undertaken according to criteria which will include the identification of risk (Brearley, 1982). Once criteria have been established it is not difficult to systematise them. What is critical is that the work on the criteria be undertaken thoroughly and be non-discriminatory. The debate over the risk of custody scales in the Probation Service is a useful example. These scales are used to target individuals who are at risk of a custodial sentence and the aim is to offer effective non-custodial packages. The scales have incorporated the research evidence that women and black people are more likely to be sent to prison at earlier points in their career than white men. By incorporating this into a risk of custody scale, the argument is that discriminatory practices are systematised and condoned. The intention here is not to rehearse the arguments for and against such scales, but to emphasise that, for example, risk of residential care scales are already a reality, but must be scrutinised for inherent discriminatory practices. Is it right to make the assumption that elderly men are less able to care for themselves than women or that certain ethnic communities provide extended family care for the elderly populations?

The example of the assessment of someone over 75 years also highlights some of the tensions which may occur, because it will have a different emphasis if it is undertaken on an annual visit from the GP to someone in their own home or if it is carried out in a hospital ward by a consultant with a limited number of beds. Also a representative of a social services department will bring to such an assessment a set of considerations other than the medical. These issues underpin the need for the person undertaking the assessment to have appropriate knowledge, qualification and status to ensure that a comprehensive and balanced assessment is produced.

Having said that, it has to be acknowledged that the use of qualified workers does have other implications. Consumers do not perceive themselves as having equal status with professionally qualified social workers. Traditionally those who are in need of the services of the statutory helping agencies are not used to being advocates and will not necessarily have the skills for asserting their needs, even if they can identify them. Thus, while the third part of the process identified above – 'Take the wishes of the individual consumer into account' – will involve all the social work skills of active listening and empathy, it will also require that the care manager be prepared to work with an advocate, chosen or appointed to mediate the client's wishes.

The outcome of the assessment

The production of an assessment and the subsequent action highlight significant changes in social work practice in community care. 'Planning concerns must be balanced. There is little point in having a comprehensive individualized assessment if the care plans all look alike. There is little point to a standardised assessment if its excessive length and privacy-invading style drives needy clients away' (Steinberg and Carter, 1984, p. 12). For example, the right to assessment for certain groups has implications for the production of an assessment document. Should the outcome of the assessment process be a document given to the consumer to enable them to negotiate their own right to services, along the lines of a prescription for spectacles? Both in the Kent scheme (Challis and Davies, 1989) and in those reviewed by Renshaw (1988) the recommendation for service delivery seems to be an important part of the assessment. However these assessments must be in part influenced, if not mediated, by an awareness of the availability or acceptability of services. While the assessment should not be limited by lack of resources, it should not raise hopes unrealistically. The outcome of an assessment where the desired services are not available may be a compromise, such as offering the limited services that are available, or postponing intervention in a case until the services become available. An outcome identified by Challis and Davies (1989) is that sometimes an appropriate assessment would be to recommend offering limited help for consumers who are suspicious of social work intervention in order to build up confidence in the system.

This wide-ranging process is significant, both for the tasks needed to be performed to complete a viable assessment and for the workload implications. It is possible to see the process as an incremental one involving a first initial assessment on the basis of whether the client fits the categories identified by the agency as being appropriate for service delivery. This might involve a simple form filling exercise. Those who are eligible are then subject to a fuller assessment on the basis of which needs are identified and service delivery requirements outlined. This second stage process would involve wide-scale consultation and include the professional opinions of others where appropriate. The results of this process could be that three documents are prepared: a detailed set of recommendations for possible service providers which would amount to a programme for action; a contract for the nature and frequency of services to be provided; and a synopsis of this which can be given to the consumer and to which reference can be made for quality assurance and review purposes.

Planning and securing the delivery of care

The third function in the process of care management is that, having identified and agreed upon the services needed in a particular case, these services are then delivered. There is of course an interim process. While the assessment is a 'stand alone' stage which should identify the needs and strengths of the individual, those who perform the task cannot operate in a vacuum. Issues which will need to be addressed include whether existing services are to be used and clients slotted into a range of existing provision, for example volunteers, a voluntary organisation and/or an independent organisation already contracted, or whether for each new client a tailor-made system can be invoked which will help to meet the identified needs. This stage marks the crucial link between large-scale service planning and individual client assessment. The wide-scale planning occurs in the production of the community care plans, which are to be both a consultative process and a means of stimulating the community. While need will be identified at a geographical level, any service planning also has to assimilate the information from each individual assessment. It is the process of securing the ser-vices on the basis of assessment which will determine whether community care is a reality for all client groups, or only some.

Implicit in the statement that services have been agreed upon is the notion that the resources, in terms of budgets, are available and there is agreement that the particular pack-age is cost-effective. The skills needed for these sets of assumptions have, to date, been required at higher manage-ment level. Budgetary devolution in care management could require that such considerations are made at service man-ager, care manager or even consumer level.

Another set of assumptions is about the range of services which might be required to meet an individual or a group of individuals' needs. The suggestion is that making use of the voluntary 'not for profit' or independent providers as well as the existing services of the statutory social services depart-ments will help to increase the range of services available. A further option in a mixed economy of care is that the statu-tory authorities develop innovative ways of providing neces-sary services which are not already part of their repertoire or are not provided by the other sectors. But, as Smale and Tuson (1990) rightly comment, 'packages of care cannot be plucked out of the ether, or out of the "community". For staff of social work and social service agencies to adopt a care-management approach to packages of care, they will have to have a range of alternatives to offer' (1990, p. 155). The question they pose about who will create the alternatives is pertinent, but the model of organisational change that Smale and Tuson advocate does not go far enough. To change an organisation to enable entrepreneurial or innovative social workers to 'do their own thing' might produce pockets of excellent practice, but it will not necessarily ensure a coherent organisational response to identified need. This requires systematic work on stimulating the voluntary and independent sector, preparing contracts and encouraging innovatory practice within social service departments. The way that packages are presented is also critical. Social workers tend to resist the model of 'off the peg' packages, suggesting that it depersonalises the process and detracts from their professional expertise, but these may be effective in ensuring that client needs are met.

Qualities of the worker who secures services

The implications for care managers, whether social workers or not, of planning and securing services in the community are that individual autonomy and professional exclusiveness may be challenged. What is needed is the ability to recognise the skills and professionalism of other colleagues, despite differences in their qualifications and experiences. A preparedness to identify the capacity of non-professionals, be they volunteer, informal carer or consumer, to provide an excellent standard of care is also essential. These qualities would be necessary in the individual undertaking the care package planning, but other qualities might be necessary in order to secure the actual provision of the services. While Smale and Tuson find that there can be no substitute for local knowledge in the identification and provision of services, Renshaw suggests that 'attitudes, enthusiasm and common sense can be at least as important as qualifications' (1988, p. 101).

If the requirement of care management in community care is for holistic, problem-focused assessments which use lateral thinking in their approach to problem solving and draw upon a wide variety of service providers, then how will this requirement be met? Having established the need for the professional social worker at the assessment stage, what are the implications for personnel at the point of securing services?

Planning and securing services requires expertise which is not always apparent within the repertoire of social workers. When the Barclay Report made recommendations about changes in approach within social work practice, there were critics who thought that some of the barriers to inter-agency collaboration were insurmountable. Webb, for instance, lists 'organisational structure, the extent and locus of worker autonomy, the divergent perceptions of the nature of the problem facing clients' (1983, p. 46) as some of the hurdles to co-operative working between statutory agencies. To that we can add a resistance to allowing voluntary agencies a share in the process because of lack of trust and professional arrogance. If the mixed economy of care provision is to be a reality, then workers need to be able to liaise with other organisations at an early stage, otherwise there will be significant barriers to the development of services.

The need to overcome such barriers is illustrated by the expressed concern of the Commission for Racial Equality (1990), who welcome the potential for the involvement of ethnic minority community groups in planning and delivering appropriate services for the needs of ethnic minority clients. The Commission argues that the contribution of such specialist groups could be both in training and in direct service provision. These sentiments are echoed by groups such as the National Schizophrenia Fellowship, who see themselves as having identified knowledge and expertise in their areas.

To provide a true mixed economy provision it is necessary to work with existing organisations, to be able to utilise existing provision. The opportunity for housing associations to provide support in the community for those with learning difficulties, or for the local association of MIND to staff drop-in facilities by working with the users of the mental health services, is apparent. The next stage is to stimulate voluntary and private or independent organisations to respond flexibly and be prepared to produce wide ranges of services. There has been no reluctance in the private sector to provide residential care for the elderly, but the provision of day care and drop-in facilities tends to be left to voluntary organisations. The issue here is obviously one of assured income, if not profit. The opportunity to devolve budgets to enable day care facilities to be funded on an economic basis might be a stimulant to the private sector. However it will require considerable vision, energy and powers of persuasion on the part of the individual responsible for stimulating the response.

A further piece of work which needs to be undertaken is the development of appropriate volunteer systems. The recruitment, training and support of volunteers within a statutory agency is a major task requiring particular skills. Traditionally social workers in local authorities have not used such support systems, although the probation service does have a history of encouraging practice in this area (Barr, 1971). Recent developments in local authorities have encouraged the establishment of posts such as volunteer organisers and the identification of tasks involved in such a post. The need for equitable status of the volunteer organiser within the organisation is essential if securing of diverse means of service delivery is to be a reality.

An obvious consequence of empowering clients is that, once the assessment has been made and agreed with the consumer, they are given the resources to negotiate their own package of care. Information will have to be made available to enable them to make decisions about the appropriateness of the package of care or the quality of the service offered. Consumers have not always been given information about the range of services available to them and in some cases they are not aware of what a particular service can offer. If you have never tasted caviar it is difficult to tell with your first mouthful if it is good or not. If you have never had a home carer it is difficult to know what she or he should be doing for you. For consumers to have a range of choices it will still be necessary for the statutory, voluntary and independent sector to be stimulated to meet needs in flexible and appropriate ways.

The implication of this part of the care management process is that a whole new set of negotiations and skills is required of the worker. An alternative is that a number of different workers are involved, each with a repertoire of skills, taking responsibility for different parts of the process. For example, to plan and secure a care package on the basis of an assessment, information about the range of services will need to be made available, consumer opinions sought and responded to. If the necessary service is not available in the statutory sector, then some form of brokerage role will need to be performed by liaising with the voluntary and independent sectors. Those delivering the services will need to be explicit about what is on offer, and the cost involved. The consumer will have an opinion on the acceptability of the package of care and the budget holder, if it is not the consumer, will make a decision about the cost-effectiveness of the package.

Monitoring the quality of care provided

As with the initial contracting of services, monitoring the quality of care might be carried out at departmental management level, but more likely it would fall to a service manager, someone with knowledge and expertise of a particular client group and with a broad overview within the organisation:

someone who could negotiate with and call to task appropriate people within their own and other organisations. The setting up of quality assurance units is a way of identifying necessary skills and expertise and providing an appropriate structure within the organisation to carry out the numerous functions. However, even where these units are operating, there are aspects of monitoring quality which have to go on at every stage in the process of care management. Yardsticks have to be designed, targets set, or other forms of measurement of quality designed and communicated to those involved in the process.

Monitoring quality is not just a matter of responding to dissatisfied customers or checking that the service provider is actually carrying out the care plan, whatever that plan might be. In arguing that such monitoring has to be effective, we also suggest that the process of monitoring and assuring the quality of service delivery involves a number of different tasks, which in their turn depend upon a range of skills and access to appropriate information. At the widest level, monitoring the quality of care means knowing that the clients whose needs are identified are offered services which meet the criteria identified by the agency for quality and quantity. To do this effectively there will need to be feedback from a variety of sources which are now considered.

Using information

Monitoring the quality and quantity of services makes specific requirements of information systems. In the first instance, information is needed from the care planning process on the packages offered and the outcomes so that the predictive skills of individual care managers can be enhanced. Obviously care managers will have their own experience of the outcomes of what they have done, but it is the sharing of this information that is critical. One important set of information which will be part of the monitoring process is a cost–benefit analysis of different forms of service.

This will require comparative data and will be part of the information sharing process. Additionally information from reviews can contribute to this and a continual review of the longer-term outcomes from the inputs will be necessary. An example of this is the debate over the role of home care services. An analysis of the actual tasks undertaken compared with the level of, for example, immobility of the recipient would help to give information not only about the number of home carers that are necessary, but also about the skills they will need to perform the tasks.

Other requirements include a database which allows for information to be provided on chosen performance indicators, that is activities or outcomes which are identified as reflecting good quality service. One such performance indicator could be that services are given to the right clients. The definition of 'right clients' is contentious and might include all consumers who are in need of a service, or are being offered one. Referral rates are important here, but they do not give the whole picture. Knowing the percentage of the population is over a certain age tells you little about the possible demand for services. More detailed knowledge about possible risk categories is needed to identify whether services are being delivered to those who require them.

The mere collection of such data does not necessarily give information about the quality of the care offered. Decisions about innovative care packages or extending the opportunities for community care are linked to some notion of what can or should be offered and to whom. They also need to be dependent upon more information than that which says simply that the package of care was offered and the individual is still in the community. To go beyond this requires some feedback from those receiving services. However surveys of current consumers' opinions do not always give you the relevant information. The issue of service delivery to ethnic minority groups highlights the fact that people who do not receive a service cannot comment on its quality, and a service which is not available to all who are in need of it is somewhat lacking in overall quality. This is not to devalue surveys of consumer opinion but to caution that they need careful consideration.

Consumer opinion

This identification of the consumers' part in the process of quality assurance is vital from a number of aspects. The first is that in identifying quality of care there has to be some notion of what is acceptable quality. To retain individuals in the community in order to avoid the cost of residential care, but at the risk of their quality of life, is counter to the principles of social work and community care. An oft-cited example of this dilemma of measuring quality is the take up of meals on wheels (Tutt, 1990). To have a measure of how many meals on wheels are being delivered is nonsensical if the meals are unappetising and are being consigned to the bin! On the other hand standards have to be appropriate. We do not have to have designer packages of care or nouvelle cuisine meals to establish quality. These become prohibitive in terms of cost, set unattainable standards and may not be any more appetizing or acceptable to the consumer. For packages of care this means that quality has to be related to the identified needs of the individual and sufficient to deal with the problems within their circumstances. This does not mean that clients with a higher expectation or standard of living should get better services, but that the services provided should be relevant to the consumer.

The task for the care manager is to ensure that consumers are allowed the opportunity both to identify their own needs and to comment on what is offered. The process of involving individuals in identifying needs and taking part in the process of assessing outcomes has its roots in community work, social planning and contract work, and there are some very real lessons to be learnt from these methods of intervention. While social workers are trained in listening skills, they need to be aware of the way their status might inhibit consumers from stating their true opinions. Also the people whose opinions are sought may come from groups within society, which are based on age (children, for example), class, race and gender, who traditionally have not been encouraged to have opinions of their own, let alone state them. The notion that members of such groups will suddenly be able to assert their opinions as individuals is unrealistic. They will need to be encouraged and assisted to speak out. Evidence from such organisations as Gingerbread and MIND indicates that, through collective support or developing necessary skills, it is possible for consumer groups to be effective, but care management will have to ensure that individuals and groups are given the necessary support and training in, for example, assertiveness, advocacy and negotiating skills.

Such support will have to recognise that individuals might well be inhibited from speaking out when the caring is provided by a family member. Those in need of the care are often acutely aware of being a drain or a demand and will at times subvert their own needs in order not to impose upon the lives of others. If the quality of care offered by family members is not appropriate, by whatever criteria, it is difficult for an individual to complain.

Advocacy

One way of addressing these issues is to have an advocate who could work with individuals, giving information, helping make their own evaluation, and encouraging them to voice their opinions. In the last analysis the advocate could speak on behalf of the consumer, especially at reviews. For the advocate to be the same individual as the care manager could cause certain role confusion and be inhibiting to the consumer. There is scope to have users' rights officers or consumer relations officers within local authority provision, to help inform all services and create a culture which is responsive to the needs and concerns of users and carers. The use of representatives of voluntary organisations, volunteers or informal carers is an obvious possibility, as is an independent advocacy scheme (Hunter, 1988). Such arrangements raise other issues of quality and quantity assurance in that there will need to be some oversight of the schemes to ensure they are properly resourced and accessible to all who require them.

Supporting providers

Recognising the demands that caring puts on the service providers is important. Home carers, for example, might be performing the same task for a number of demanding individuals several times a day. No matter how strong the motivation, it is important that the demands are recognised and opportunities for offloading some of the pressures are offered. This becomes even more critical when volunteers are recruited to provide a part of a particular package. Acknowledging the strain of simple tasks with highly dependent or demanding individuals helps the carer to cope. For all informal carers, it is also a case of recognising the personal investment they have made in the caring, the complex emotions that might be involved, and the support and respite needed to enable them to continue caring without resentment and reluctance.

Contract compliance

In discussing the care planning process it was noted that it becomes the blueprint for the services offered, the basis of the contract both in terms of services and costing. As such it sets out the levels of service, contact time and resources. To ensure that the organisation providing the service, whether private, voluntary or statutory, keeps to the terms of the contract some form of contract compliance is required. The significance for the front line worker will be to ensure that monitoring can take place. Will it involve observation of the actual interactions with consumers or merely a form filling exercise on the part of the person or organisation delivering the service, confirming that certain tasks were completed by various individuals at particular times? One possibility would be that each consumer be allocated a diary sheet to be completed by a visiting volunteer, community nurse or whoever else it might be. The care manager may then have to check attendance against agreed contact levels. However all that would be monitored here is the quantity of service; the consumer would be given no opportunity to comment on the quality.

It is also within contract compliance that the issue of race equality can be addressed. 'The provider's response to the purchaser's requirements should include provision of services adequate for and appropriate to the needs of all ethnic groups being served, and information about race equality performance in service delivery' (CRE, 1990b). Within the provision of the Race Relations Act, local authorities are charged with eliminating discrimination on the basis of race from their services. It will be incumbent upon them in the community care provisions to ensure that all services are ethnically sensitive, whoever is providing them.

It may be that responsibility for monitoring does not fall to the individual care manager. Indeed Steinberg and Carter (1983) indicate real difficulties if the care manager also has to monitor quality. Such difficulties may arise if care managers have to comment critically on the service provided by another part of their own organisation. Also if a critical evaluation of the quality of the service of other organisations is made then the suggestion is that the services of the evaluating agency must be beyond reproach. The provision of an accredited list might meet some of these difficulties, but this would need to be effectively monitored and the criteria made public. Finally the care management process is in itself a form of service and as such needs to be subject to quality assurance. It is obviously inappropriate for care managers to be the people to assess their own performance.

Review of client needs

The process of review is not new to social workers already
familiar with it through fostering placements, adult placements, or children in residential care. In community care the
purpose of care management is to devise packages of care to
retain individuals in the community and the effectiveness of
these needs regular review. Studies of the Kent scheme
(Challis and Davies, 1989) and parallel schemes in America
(Steinberg and Carter, 1983) claim that care management
may provide more effective intervention in long-term cases,
but the reality is that the circumstances of these particular
clients are not necessarily going to improve. In fact in many
situations, particularly those involving elderly people, ultimately a deterioration is anticipated. Review therefore means
ensuring that the services provided are meeting needs as they
change. It also means responding to situations where services
need to be changed, replaced, modified or terminated.

The care manager has to ensure that review processes are
effective. Initially a programme for reviews needs to be
established. This demands a flexibility of response, but the
obvious first requirement is that a review should be written
into the care plans. Reviews at regular intervals, that is, a
fixed point review, would ensure a regular opportunity to
evaluate the services being offered, which would provide
ongoing support or maintenance to those who are providing
the services. This is particularly significant where the client is
providing his or her own care plans. However we have
established that circumstances change over time. These
changes include the physical deterioration of those requiring
care and a lessening of the ability of the carers, especially
informal carers, to tolerate the new circumstances.

How the review is carried out is also important. An effective review could involve the same processes as the initial
assessment, with input from all involved in the situation.
This has been termed the process reassessment (Steinberg
and Carter, 1983) rather than review. The process could be a

fairly routinised collection of information for the fixed point review, but might need more comprehensive information gathering and re-evaluation if it is an 'exceptions' review, that is one brought about by a specific change in circumstances. A more limited review would be an update on the delivery of services.

There are points to consider about the review stage which have implications for the other parts of the care management process as we have described it. The first is that it will give information about the effectiveness of service delivery and as such will feed into the processes of monitoring quality. It will also give feedback on the level and frequency of services which will feed into the aggregated systems of service provision and will have implications for resources and budgets. Finally implicit in the function of review is that it involves an evaluation of services obtained through care management as well as the services of the care manager. Consequently it brings the whole process of care management full circle in that it is an evaluation of the initial assessment itself. To this end, while it would be the care manager's task to orchestrate regular reviews and respond to the need for an exceptions review, there is also a role for advocates in the review process. They could ensure that the views of the consumer are heard and request reviews if they have not been initiated by the care manager.

The need for such a review process is obvious for those who are receiving services, but there is also an argument for identifying review processes for situations which have been assessed, but were identified as not being in need of care management at the time. The system of annual assessment of those over 75 will allow these individuals opportunities to have their circumstances reviewed and to be offered care if appropriate. Such a safeguard needs to be available to other groups. In particular, those cases where clients had previously been coping, but circumstances have now deteriorated, require the assurance that early attention will be given to their needs.

The role of the care manager

At the beginning of this chapter we looked at two sets of components for care management, both of which involved a range of tasks. They identified similar tasks and, these having been analysed in some detail, it is apparent that while the process of care management in community care requires that all these tasks be performed, they do not all have to be performed by the same individual, the care manager. Indeed it may not be desirable, from both the professional and the organisational viewpoint, for the care manager to do everything. The appointment of a care manager is critical to the whole process of care management, but to ensure that this individual is able to manage that process effectively some tasks may have to be delegated. This is not to minimise those tasks. In fact part of the necessity for delegating them is to ensure that they are performed to the highest possible standards by individuals with appropriate skills.

In the above sections we have suggested that the identification of need, securing services and monitoring quality all depend upon significant input from other workers, even if they are not fully taken over by them. Preparing an assessment and undertaking reviews are the responsibility of one individual, although they draw on other sources for information. What then does the care manager do? For the care management process to function effectively the care manager will prepare the assessment and act upon it. Alternatively s/he may receive a full assessment, prepared by another worker, and implement it. S/he will certainly retain contact with the client while the necessary work is done to secure services and will have a vital role to play in negotiating the introduction of services, whoever provides them. It is unlikely that a whole package of resources will be delivered at the door of, for example, an elderly person on the same day without any introductions or phased implementation. In some situations it may be possible for the care manager to maintain a minimal role once services are operating effectively. However we have to acknowledge that, with many situations, the process will not be one of clearly defined separate phases. Assessments will be incremental and services requirements will change over time, because other needs are identified, or the client becomes more confident in the community and requests more or less assistance or, of course, if the situation deteriorates and a review is necessary.

In these situations we have pointed out that the process of care management is a circular one and that many of the tasks and indeed the personnel are interdependent. However what is also clear is that even in this interdependence one worker has to retain an overview of the situation, to ensure that all the other resources, human, financial and otherwise, are used to best effect, that the identified services are provided to an adequate standard, and that changes in client circumstances are quickly noted.

In addition, the major implication of the mixed economy of welfare provision is that, where different people do perform different tasks, they will not necessarily be professionally qualified social workers, or indeed social workers at all. Bamford (1990) predicts on the basis of the Griffiths Report that the skills needed will not be specific to social work and indeed, this prediction is fulfilled in *Caring for People*, which is quite specific on the point: 'It is not essential that the same manager should undertake all these tasks for a particular client but a clearly identified individual should be designated for each function. The Government does not wish to be prescriptive about the background from which the care manager should be drawn' (Department of Health, 1989, para.3.3.4).

Organisation of the task

Renshaw's overview (1988) of existing schemes in both Britain and America also emphasises that the organisation of care management and related schemes may involve personnel other than professionally qualified social workers and can involve the use of workers according to different organisational models. The overview given above indicates that there is a lot of scope within the care management process for different functions to be performed by different workers, and we now need to consider the range of different organisational models. These can include specialist care managers, multi-disciplinary teams and individuals carrying a mix of care management and mainstream workloads. What are the implications of these models?

Specialist care manager. This model would require one worker, appropriately qualified, to carry a *workload* focusing specifically on the tasks related to care management. S/he would carry no cases other than those needing a care management approach, but would undertake a number of tasks related to the care management process. In many ways this would seem to be an ideal, in that such specialists have the opportunity to develop skills and identify networks to enable them to perform the necessary tasks effectively.

In terms of the management of such a system there are a number of factors to be considered. The first is the need to identify the tasks that would constitute the *workload* involved in care management. A means of assessing this workload needs to be developed which would require more than logging the number of cases. The tasks include designing, organising and purchasing services and, as Renshaw observes, 'It is undoubtedly true that care managers in care in the community schemes are very busy, very active and generally work longer hours than stipulated in their contracts of employment' (1988, p. 102). This overwork comes in situations where generally workers in care management schemes have had smaller caseloads (Challis and Davies, 1989; Beardshaw, 1990). All-in-one workers may well widen their workload and take on overload which ultimately will lead to a diminution in the quality of service and worker burn-out (Vickery, 1977; Glastonbury, Bradley and Orme, 1987). The obverse is also true: 'The size of the caseload will influence the range of tasks that an individual care manager is able to carry out and the amount of time he or she is able to devote to each' (Renshaw, 1988, p. 87). The necessity for monitoring therefore becomes paramount at the individual worker level. It is needed to ensure not only that the necessary tasks are being done but also that the worker is not attempting to do too much. This measure of 'too much' of course is dependent on some notion of what can be achieved by an individual in care management schemes and how this compares with workloads carried by others operating in mainstream social work.

Apart from the amount of work involved the specialist care manager role might have implications for the nature of the intervention and the objective of care management. If such an objective in a mixed economy of welfare is to meet individual needs by a variety of interventions, then there may be less need for the specialist counselling skills identified as the social worker's expertise (BASW, 1977; Barclay, 1982). However American studies have found that the employment of professional social workers as specialist care managers can at times subvert the aims of the scheme. For example, professionally qualified care managers in America were more prone to identify the need for and indeed carry out counselling rather than engage in co-ordination, carrying out practical tasks and other work necessary for care management (Caragonne, 1980). Part of the reason for this may be to do with individual worker satisfaction, but it may also be related to the finding that professionals were reluctant to take on extra work which did not accord with their training and status (Pelletier, 1983).

This may not be stubborn resistance to the implementation of new methods of intervention. The implication for workers in the Kent study (Challis and Davies, 1989) is apparent in the categorisation of the way social workers used their time within the broad care management scheme. The findings, that the greatest proportion of time was spent on client-related activity, may be encouraging to social workers until they discover that this was only 34.8 per cent of the care manager's time and some of that was spent in arranging services rather than direct contact with clients. This gives a clear indication that the way social workers become involved in care management will be significantly different from mainstream direct service provision.

The care manager in the multi-disciplinary team. In this model the social worker becomes the manager and in effect care management becomes the system by which social work and other inputs, the planning and allocation of services, are organised. This process can involve setting up packages of care, parts of which may be provided by other professionals, volunteers, relatives and representatives of the voluntary agencies. A central figure has to be the person who co-ordinates all of these activities and ensures service provision for the individual consumer, that is the care manager. However centrality does not necessarily mean that this person makes the major input in terms of worker time. This draws attention to the need to work as a team, coping with members from different professional backgrounds who are operating as care managers. An example of this involves the following circumstances: a care package for a 65-year-old lady with a learning difficulty and a degree of physical handicap who was living in a warden-controlled flat included input from two MENCAP support workers, a private contract cleaner and contact with the warden of the accommodation. A social worker oversaw the arrangements in this situation, but did not have the greatest amount of contact. Also the woman in question had friends and other supporters who could well have negotiated the package for her, and had oversight of it.

The worker with a mixed workload. In many situations the current legislative prescription is likely to produce situations where care management is provided for selected client groups or for individuals with particular needs within those client groups. This may mean that, rather than specialist care managers or specialist teams being established, staff will have to handle a workload which involves some cases requiring the skills and activities relating to care management, and other cases with a traditional mainstream one-to-one contact model. Because of the demands of care management, this is probably the least attractive and least efficient method of organising the service, as the following example shows. A social worker had half of her time allocated to a pilot care management scheme. She was expected to provide a brokerage service for the scheme, that is, finding the means to provide identified services. Initially this involved drawing on contacts and networks already established, but, as the number of packages increased, resources became stretched and she had to utilise other skills and networks. She had an increasing sense that she was using up more than half of her time, but as there was no agreed ceiling for what should be done in the time available it was difficult for her to argue the case. Apart from the disadvantages for the individual worker in this example there are also resource implications. Because she continued to try and do as much as possible, there was no realistic assessment of the resource needs of either the care management scheme or the mainstream social work which was the other part of her job.

Fundamental to much of the discussion is the assumption that there are specific tasks within care management that can be separated and allocated. Having established this, it also becomes clear that a monitoring system is necessary to enable service managers to ensure that individual workers from the same agency, or from different agencies performing different parts of the care management function, have equitable workloads. Such concerns are about, for example, whether the process of identifying people in need demands as much time and professional input as monitoring the quality of care provided.

Monitoring input becomes more critical when workers involved in particular cases come from different agencies, either voluntary or independent, because it is necessary to identify the cost to the particular agency and to calculate the realistic cost of the package of care. In a purchaser–provider split the costing of services also becomes relevant to all worker input.

Summary

In this chapter we have taken a comprehensive view of both the process of care management and the function of care managers within that process. Throughout we have tried to build on the discussion of the previous chapter and indicate where issues of discriminatory practice might be critical. In doing this we have focused deliberately upon the front line social worker and have attempted to link tasks involved in care management with the skills already demonstrated by these workers.

This has raised two issues: what are the new and different skill requirements of the care management process, and are the skills required for care management the prerogative of the professionally qualified social worker? In our analysis we conclude that there are many skills in care management which are consistent with social work values and expertise; in particular those involved in assessment, with identifying needs at the level of the individual and introducing services, whoever provides them, to the person in need have been identified as requiring social work expertise. Ongoing review, intervening on behalf of individuals and aspects of all the care management process which involve interpersonal skills are also in line with much traditional social work activity. Other functions, such as stimulating potential service providers, monitoring quality at an organisational level, costing packages of care and negotiating contracts with others as service providers require a different set of skills.

Workers in other organisations, voluntary and statutory, or in other parts of social services may well have these skills, but in acknowledging the additional functions we have also raised the issue of where in the organisation the responsibility for the care management process rests. This leads us to consider the management of care management. This involves organisational responsibility for ensuring that the systems are there to enable effective care management: liaising with the community, quality assurance units, volunteer organisers, advocacy systems and so on. More fundamentally we find that, at the individual worker level, the organisational level and at inter-agency level there is a significant task to be performed in ensuring the effective delivery of service. This effectiveness is a matter of ensuring not just that tasks are performed, but that the individuals performing them, whatever their background, have the appropriate levels of work to ensure best professional practice, that is, that the workload involved in the task is managed. The need for workload measurement and management is acknowledged as critical, not just for the provision of effective service but for the realistic costing of services. Hence in the next chapter we consider the tasks involved in managing all aspects of the care management process, the role of the front line manager.

5

Managing Diversity: Management Responsibilities of Care Management

Introduction

Care management in community care is to do with empowering individuals. The right to assessment, the involvement of consumers in making decisions about services and the monitoring of service delivery is said to give them more control over the process. However it is apparent that other factors are involved in empowerment. In Chapter 2 we acknowledged that access to and control over resources, whether those are services or budgets, is a significant aspect of empowerment.

Whether care management in community care achieves empowerment of individuals and communities seems to be integrally linked with the organisation of service delivery. One possible interpretation of recommendations of *Caring for People* (Department of Health, 1989) is that, if they are laid upon existing social service provision they will merely impose organisational structures and control on geographical areas and the voluntary sector. The planning process will become a bureaucratic exercise at chief officer level. A more positive outcome is that within the process of care management the intervention of the care manager to identify needs, locate services and monitor the service delivery is in itself, as the name implies, a management function and as such can be used to allow individualisation of services and consumer control of resources. If this is to be a reality, there are implications for the way that care management itself is organised and the framework in which it is managed. Social workers have been managers for some time, both self-managers and managers of individuals and families. They have also been the subject of management themselves.

Management and care management

Care management brings a new dimension to the social worker as manager. While the unitary approach to social work, the acknowledgement that individuals functioned within and are influenced by family, neighbourhood and other systems (Pincus and Minahan, 1973) prepared social workers for focusing on targets other than the individual as an appropriate point for intervention, it did not involve the substantial responsibilities which care management can demand of the individual worker. Recruiting others to deliver the service, not just at the level of domiciliary or home care support, but by handing over completely the face-to-face involvement with the consumer to someone totally outside the organisational structure, that is, someone who is not accountable within that agency, is a new challenge. Social workers have generally resisted 'handing over' cases even to their own colleagues. In this context, the idea that social workers might make the decision to hand over control completely to the carer, or indeed the consumer, seems even more unlikely. However this is a possible, if remote, implication of care management. Social services departments could become units of self-regulating care managers working with a group of brokers, negotiating with service providers and perhaps supported by finance specialists to assist with the cost–benefit analysis of the packages of care. The implication of such a scenario is that the need for the traditional team leader, the front line manager, could disappear.

The reality is that, either because of fierce resistance to change in job allocations or role definitions, or because they perform a necessary function within the process of providing care, the layer of front line managers will not disappear from the organisations but that their function will change considerably. Already in the probation service the senior probation officer has assumed a more administrative role, usually carrying no caseload, but negotiating with courts, communities and the voluntary sector for the provision of services, as well as retaining responsibility for the standard of service provided by individual probation officers. Similar developments have occurred in the changing roles and tasks of nurse managers and head teachers as managers in the current reorganisation of public services.

Discussions to date suggest that there will be a continuing need for a form of front line management in the development of care management in community care, and that the functions to be performed will be critical to the successful implementation of schemes. There is less consensus about how organisations can achieve the changes necessary for effective service delivery. Hadley and Young advocate that these changes will involve new structures requiring 'local, integrated teams; increasing devolution of decision making; the active use of projects to explore new ways of working in the community, as well as opening the agency to user influence; and later the testing and implementation of local financial management' (1990, p. ii). This will ensure that the agency responds to the demands of, and meets the characteristics identified by, the Audit Commission (1986) as necessary for successful initiatives in community care. However the suggestion by Hadley and Young that this can best be achieved by a radical and imposed reorganisation of agency staff, and can be reinforced by keeping those staff in a permanent state of change, appears somewhat draconian. When the Hadley and Young model has been applied in other areas the ensuing staff morale has been a block to, rather than an enhancement of, communication and co-operation.

This approach is contrasted and complemented by that of Smale and Tuson (1990), who argue that for community care to be effective there is the need for small, relatively autonomous units which can work more closely with consumers. For this to be achieved requires the change in orientation *of* teams as well as *for* teams. For example, if teams are to bring about the necessary practice changes for true community care, or in their terms community social work, then teams themselves will have to undergo change. This will enable them to make local decisions and partnerships and not be locked into hierarchical and bureaucratic processes. Rather than this occurring through structures being imposed from above in the way that Hadley and Young advocate, workers will have to be innovative and flexible despite the wider organisation. Rather than reorganisation causing unhappiness and dissent among workers, they suggest that innovations at team level might cause tensions within the management system but lead to greater worker satisfaction.

This dichotomy of views on how to create the environment in which to implement care management highlights two concerns which will be explored. One is the effective organisation of workers involved in care management. The other is leadership of the care management team.

Organisation for care management

The consideration of how to organise for care management is closely related to the debate in Chapter 4 about what tasks need to be performed and by whom. The permutations for the organisation are numerous and of course each has implications for the role and tasks of the individual who has immediate line management responsibility for them.

If agencies elect to have specialised care managers working primarily on the task of overseeing the services to the consumer, then such individuals could be part of a specialist team of care managers working with the same client group. This specialist team does not have to be collected in the same geographical location; they could be decentralised and organised on patch systems so that the task of working with community resources becomes more of a reality. If this distribution does occur, what models could be utilised in the organisation of 'patch' teams? There is the possibility of having patch teams of care managers who are working with different consumer groups. This is an unlikely response to the policy initiatives which urge the implementation of care management for certain client groups only, but it may be a pointer to future organisation. A more likely outcome is that specialist care managers will be part of an interdisciplinary group, but one in which other individuals from the same discipline are not working to a care management model.

Challis and Davis seem to be arguing for some form of specialist model when they note that 'an attempt to enable staff from an area team to work with a few community care cases, while continuing with their usual workload for the rest of the time, did not prove successful' (1989, p. 228). They concluded that this model has implications for workers particularly in relation to parity of workloads. Their findings, that care management does increase expertise and commitment to client groups and that there is a greater willingness to implement community care for clients in longer-term need, are significant. If care management is not introduced for all client groups simultaneously, then there will be disparity in the allocation of resources whether those resources be budgets or direct worker time. On the other hand specialist care managers may not necessarily be the norm. Agencies could elect to introduce an element of care management for all workers. The introduction of this method of organising the work would depend upon client need and each and any worker might therefore be involved in developing packages of care.

Finally, if the care management process is to be truly multi-disciplinary, then the organisation of individual care managers as workers with responsibility for brokers, service providers and others, including representatives of statutory services such as health and housing and volunteers, carers and consumers, is required. Each care manager becomes part of a mini-team or working group. A cluster of such individual care managers could be accountable to someone within the organisation who performs the next level of management tasks. The critical question is, what are these tasks?

It may be possible to identify sets of tasks which can be carried out by individual managers. It is also important to consider organisational change which would split the tasks between individual managers. Initially attention should be given to whether it is appropriate for them to be performed at the level of front line manager at all. If *care management* is the management of the intervention and activity with clients, then *service management* is the total oversight of that process, and this oversight, if it is to be effective in facilitating the operation of the total process of care management, has to be comprehensive. Is it realistic to expect that the same person should perform all the tasks required of front line management? Do these tasks require a social worker in the role of service manager? The same questions that have been asked about the role of care manager can be asked about service managers.

This questioning has not yet occurred within the personal social services in connection with care management, although, historically, reorganisation after the report of the Seebohm committee did raise such issues (Bamford, 1990). Significantly the debate is taking place in the probation service in response to proposed policy changes. The Green Paper, *Supervision and Punishment in the Community: A framework for action* is quite specific about management implications: 'If the individual probation officer has a more complex task in devising and running supervision schemes for offenders, correspondingly greater demands will be placed on senior and chief officers, as managers of the probation system. . . . There will be a greater need to monitor the outcome of supervision, and to evaluate the effectiveness – and the cost – of different approaches' (Home Office, 1990 para.3.6).

At chief officer level there is an explicit statement that people with management experience in other fields might be appointed (para.5.23). The need for training and reshaping the management role is identified (para.9.20), and some indication of what senior probation officers (front line managers) are to do is given in discussion about the need to achieve balance between reducing management grades to encourage local initiatives and appointing sufficient numbers of managers to provide close oversight, at the risk of smothering creativity and limiting local flexibility. As for front line workers (basic grade probation officers), a number of key functions are identified: the need to manage resources, organise their own time and workloads and draw effectively on the resources and skills of others around them and to motivate any staff under their direct control (para.9.15). This gives some fairly clear indications of the thinking behind the role of front line manager in the newly developing structures in probation and it is possible that similar trends will develop in other personal social services.

The tasks to be done

Whatever system of care management is to be implemented it is unlikely, indeed it is undesirable, that the scenario of self-regulating care managers outlined at the beginning of the chapter should become a reality. Even if care managers do acquire within the tasks they perform a more managerial function, there is always the need for support, supervision and accountability. These functions have been the justification of organising social work into teams, and Tom Douglas's critique (1983) of the team as a working group highlights the way that the processes which occur within groups are help-ful. If teams and working groups have to have a leader, as a manager that leader of a working group has a significant role to fulfil, not just for the team members but also for the organisation.

The tasks performed by front line management in social work can be identified as emanating from two sources, the agency or organisation which is providing a service for the clients, and the group of workers who constitute the team. The agency requires that an identified person is responsible for: allocation of work; accountability for budgets; monitor-ing and evaluation; collation of information; quality assur-ance; other day-to-day decisions; team development and supervision of individual staff. The group of workers will require that a work group leader provides: co-ordination and review of work; opportunities to reflect on practice; opportunities for the dissemination of ideas and innovations in practice; opportunities for peer support and encourage-ment; attention to individual welfare and development. For the management of care management there are further sets of imperatives which are, in the first instance, to do with implementing new systems and managing change, but are also to do with specific aspects of operating a care manage-ment scheme. It is useful therefore to compare the two sets of tasks. A way of analysing these tasks is to consider not only the requirements of different parts of the system but also the process that has to be managed. In earlier chapters we have identified the stages that have to be undertaken in care management. In Table 5.1 we present a comparison of ways in which managing care management, which we have called service management, might proceed.

What is highlighted by the comparison is that some tasks and duties remain constant for the manager, but there are also extra interventions that the policy changes will require. As with so many aspects of the current changes in policy, it is possible to argue that the skills and professional knowledge required of service managers do not differ widely from

Table 5.1   *Front line management responsibilities*

Current responsibilities	Service management
Systems for receiving work into the organisation	Systems for stimulating consumer knowledge of the services
Decisions about service offered in the light of statute and policy	Decisions about whether this is a suitable case for care management
Initial allocation of the case to worker for intervention	Allocation of the care manager
Monitoring of the overall workload of the front line worker to inform allocation decisions	Analysis of the package of care: (a) Is it realistic and workable? (b) Does it meet the criteria for keeping the client in the community? (c) Is it value for money?
Allocation decision; intervention to cease, continue with the same worker or be allocated to different worker	Contracting of care package
Allocation of key worker Supervising the worker's involvement in the case in the light of: (a) professional social work knowledge (b) policy guidelines on risk, etc. (c) knowledge of the demands of the workers overall workload	Overseeing the work which includes: (a) acknowledging the overall workload (b) receiving information about levels of intervention by all involved (c) carrying out periodic reviews.

existing requirements. However this can only be the starting-point. Just as many parts of the care management process need not be carried out by the same individual, so the management responsibilities implicit in the organisation of community care do not have to be fulfilled by the same individual.

Managing care management

The first major shift is that there is a right to be assessed. This is supported by an expectation that potential consumers will be made aware of the availability of services. Traditionally social work agencies have been reluctant to 'sell their wares'. This reluctance stems from a number of different sources but a disincentive in recent years has been the reality that social work agencies have not had the resources to cope with the demand that could be made upon them. Front line managers who have been grappling with prioritising workloads and imposing workload ceilings are being asked to ensure a non-discriminatory service delivery, and in some situations a universal right to assessment.

The identification of needs, co-operating and negotiating with other professionals such as those in health and housing, liaising with the voluntary and private sectors, the provision of services within the statutory sector, quality assurance and receipt of complaints are all activities which need to be carried out in order for the care management process to function. They do not necessarily have to be performed by the care manager. It has already been argued in Chapter 4 that if the care manager is going to be a front line worker within the organisation then it is inappropriate for some of these tasks to be left for individual negotiation. To do so would have enormous implications for individual workloads and lead to the possibility of duplication of activity within the organisation.

The tasks of stimulating the voluntary sector, encouraging diversification in the non-residential care sector and entering into partnership with both voluntary and independent sectors could be undertaken by a person with a specific brief, sometimes identified as a broker. Organisations will need to identify at what management level this role should operate. Is the brokerage task equal in demand and complexity to the care manager or is there an argument for saying that as a representative of the organisation they ought to be appointed at team or even area level?

Quality assurance could also demand a different set of skills. In one sense, quality assurance at the individual level should not be new to social work managers. The professional responsibility of worker and team leader is to ensure, through the process of supervision, that clients are offered best professional social work practice. In care management the complexity comes when the overseeing authority has to operate quality assurance not just of its own staff but of staff and services provided by other agencies. This may be possible through a system of contract compliance which could ensure levels of contact and provision of services. But service delivery is also concerned with issues of professional practice and the quality of the relationship of workers and consumers. This becomes difficult when services are being provided by volunteers and informal carers.

Essentially we can identify a number of layers to the process of care management, all of which need to have some form of co-ordinated management to ensure that tasks are performed and that there are no gaps in services. As the final responsibility for providing services where they do not exist lies with local authority social service departments, this oversight and management will rest with an employee of that organisation.

This is the reality of an interdisciplinary team in community care. Table 5.2 makes no assumptions about hierarchy, it seeks to clarify the functions which have to be managed to ensure that at the point of need the services are delivered. It will consist of people with different functions within the organisation, including social workers, occupational therapists and workers from other settings, voluntary or independent. Who will manage all these aspects? While some voluntary organisations may well be able to provide the necessary supervision of workers, will the same standard be available in the independent sector? How will reviews occur and what are the sanctions if standards are not being met?

Table 5.2   *Functions to be managed*

Service provision	Care management process	Management role
Family	Broker	
Neighbours		
Volunteers	Assessment Volunteer organiser	
Voluntary organisations	Purchasing —— Advocate	Service manager
Independent sector	Review —— Quality assurance	
Health service		
Local authority Social services		

The challenge of managing care management

This analysis of the additional tasks within the management of care management begins to highlight some of the challenges and potential conflicts for the front line manager which need further exploration.

Allocating workloads

The task of allocating work has always been a vital one for the front line manager, but the complexities of such a task are increased when considering the management function in care management. We have given the role of team manager in allocating workloads detailed consideration elsewhere (Glastonbury, Bradley and Orme, 1987). The responsibility of the manager is not to attempt to achieve detailed precision in the measuring of workloads, but to ensure that workloads are managed equably (Orme, 1988).

To achieve this in the management of care management means having clear definitions of the particular roles that need to be performed. It also means having some sense of the parity between tasks and taking the responsibility for allocating resources. This process becomes complex when the same tasks can be performed by workers with different qualifications and from different organisations. A further complication is seen when the nature of the tasks varies widely. For example the equating of the care manager role which can involve contact with demanding clients, with the brokerage role which might involve liaison with receptive organisations and agencies, needs some careful balancing.

Budgetary devolution

A major new function for front line managers linked to workload management is the budgetary aspect of costing services and possible virement of budgets between different sections. The front line manager will become involved in actual accounting functions. This will include monitoring packages of care against cost-effectiveness criteria and will inevitably involve decisions about priorities. Budgets will be finite and front line managers will need to be prepared to resolve the conflicts of competing demands. Refining packages to fit in with price may also be a function of managing individual care managers.

Managing the specialist

The responsibility for managing workers who are providing operations at a highly specialised level will bring about conflicts of management responsibility over professional decisions. The process of assessment as described in Chapter 4 is a highly complex and professional task. This task will be informed by the opinions and expertise of others, including those from different disciplines as well as carers and consumers. Also it is probable that in devising packages of care a certain amount of balancing of risks will need to be undertaken by the care manager, either on a long-term or short-term basis. Intervening in this level of expertise will not be an easy task. However it will be a function of front line management to vet the package of care, not only because decisions will be linked to budget allocation, but also because there is the need to assure the quality of all the services being offered, including the quality of the assessment. At some future point the manager may also be called upon to investigate a complaint as part of quality assurance. The dilemma here is to acknowledge the expertise of the care manager and allow a level of professional autonomy while retaining overall responsibility for the provision of the service.

Quality assurance

All staff responsible for service delivery will be subject to quality assurance monitoring. Quality assurance will not just be to do with the level of service in terms of hours of home care or time spent at a day centre, but will involve monitoring the nature of the service offered and the quality of the relationship. If a consumer complains about the care manager it will be the front line manager's responsibility to assess the situation. This means supervising work, but could also involve staff appraisal and disciplinary issues. In many ways this brings front line managers into the forefront of staffing matters. Ironically this aspect of management will challenge the assumption of personal autonomy which has persisted in the casework ethos of social services, and which has been highlighted as a necessary strength of the assessment process. The manager will need to be close enough to the worker to be able to ascertain what standard of service is being offered, but will also need to retain a professional distance to enable appropriate intervention if the standard of service is not appropriate. This explicit managerial responsibility will formalise a situation which has been implicit in social work management but perhaps has not been clarified. It is important that it not only fulfils an inspectorial function but can enable workers to improve their level of service.

Quality assurance becomes more complex when services are provided by different workers and, at times, different organisations. The front line manager will have to invoke the best judicial skills to intervene in situations where the assessment has been undertaken and the needs identified, but the complaint is that the package has not been delivered. This may be because services are not available, are available but because of worker inefficiency have not been delivered, or the line manager him or herself has ruled that the particular package of care is too costly.

A final complication for front line managers with quality control responsibilities arises when the package of care has been set up by the consumer or indeed when the consumer or informal carer is the sole service provider. While the care manager will have a watching brief it will be for the front line manager to have the final say in decision making. It could be argued that front line managers should not have responsibility for assuring the quality of packages of care not provided by social service departments, that empowerment means allowing consumers to make mistakes. Examples of people with learning difficulties and the elderly suffering abuse or neglect are the stuff of media headlines (as the Beverley Lewis case highlighted), but they also reflect the risks involved in community care strategies.

Complaints procedures

A related development is the codifying of a complaints procedure. This can be seen as the extension of work that has been developing over the last few years on consumerism and empowerment within the social services, but the refinement suggested in *Caring for People* (Department of Health, 1989) demands a different set of processes from the current arrangements. Even if a specialist complaints officer or team exists, careful negotiations with the voluntary sector will be needed. Organisations such as MIND and CRE have to date acted as advocates and pressure groups for some users of social services and require more than just forums for hearing the complaints; they also need the conditions for a dialogue to ensue about the best way to meet the demands.

Front line managers will be required to negotiate at a local level to ascertain good communication systems. They may also be required to investigate complaints against workers whose work they have had responsibility for supervising. Such complaints may come from independent advocates, but if advocacy is performed by workers within the social services agencies on behalf of consumers, then the complaints may well be lodged by one worker within the organisation against the other. The skills needed in these circumstances seem close to the qualities of Solomon!

Monitoring service delivery

A further significant function within the management of care management is monitoring services provided and identifying patterns of demand. The purpose of this is twofold. The first would be to ensure that costly service delivery could be avoided. Where a common demand becomes apparent then identifying the means to meet this at other than the individual level would avoid duplication of activity and allow for economies of scale. The second purpose is to identify the gaps in the service and to 'retain the ability to act as direct service providers, if other forms of service provision are unforthcoming or unsuitable' (Department of Health, 1989, para.3.4.11). This purchaser–provider split has implications for the front line manager, not least because theoretically they are separate tasks. It is apparent that the overall function of provider of services will have to be taken on board at the level of the total organisation because of the resource implications both in terms of budgets and staffing levels. There is also a need for the front line manager to organise the provision of a particular service, whether that be a group of locally recruited volunteers or a specialist counselling service provided by a group of appropriately trained social workers. At the same time s/he may be negotiating with local voluntary or independent groups to provide a day care facility for which the need has been identified.

The future for management in care management

Coulshed (1990) found that social work managers have a responsibility for directing, managing and supervising staff. These three processes aim to ensure long-term planning, organisation and support in the professional role. The above analysis of the additional tasks involved in managing care management and the conflicts inherent in the role if it is performed by one individual suggests that new models of management may need to be introduced. Such models will challenge some traditional assumptions about social work management such as the following.

1. All line management functions for a particular worker have to be carried out by one individual. We have identified that the range of skills needed for the management function incorporate: information technology including the collecting and aggregating of data; personnel skills including staff appraisal and disciplinary matters; organisational skills including liaising with a variety of individuals and agencies; entrepreneurial skills which involve stimulating service providers to be innovative; and public relation skills which involve publicising the services available and dealing with customer complaints. All these are in addition to the traditional skills of enabling and giving feedback, advice and direction on the professional task.

2. All line management functions have to be carried out by individuals with a social work qualification. The above list of skills indicates that many are not usually taught on social work courses, although they may be creeping into social work management courses. Also the growing number of social workers undertaking Masters in Business Administration (MBA) or other management courses suggests that the need for skills other than the traditional ones is already recognised.

Is the way forward therefore to have a range of different managers with different backgrounds providing the various functions for the individual care manager? This hardly seems feasible at the level of front line manager. It would lead to an enormous amount of the care manager's time being spent in consultation and might well lead to conflicting information and feedback. Also there would be issues of confidentiality. If the quality control manager was concerned about the service being offered by a particular care manager, would she or he have the right to information from the manager providing the supervision of the professional task? It is true that information about the client and levels of intervention should already be widely available, but what is not generally available is the information about content of supervision sessions. Can a worker be held responsible if s/he is acting on advice, guidance or even instruction from the line manager? How much influence would the resource manager have over the content of the package of care or indeed the level of worker intervention in individual cases?

At the beginning of this chapter we indicated that there were two sets of demands on the function of management and that these demands helped to clarify the role of the front line manager. In care management we have found that not only will the tasks of the manager increase, but there will also be a change in areas of responsibility, budgetary decisions being the obvious example of this. Service managers, therefore, have to offer all the front line management functions, which are to do with meeting the needs of the consumer and ensuring the quality of service delivery. This, at times, will involve issues of authority across agency boundaries and responsibility for monitoring services provided by other agencies. More importantly, this manager would have responsibility for the care tasks which are so crucial for the development of staff and the relief of stress. Nurturing the team or unit of organisation, whatever its composition, providing opportunities for sharing ideas and developing strategies in the context of community care, and identifying the necessary staff development and training resources to fulfil these, would be essential functions of this level of management. There is no doubt that the service manager has to be a front line manager, working closely with the care managers. What is questionable is whether one person can take responsibility for all these tasks. Care management might require that the functions are split between different service managers, or that the ratio of service managers to care managers is greater than in the traditional team arrangements. From our point of view this highlights the need for evaluation of workloads at all levels. All service management functions have to include a responsibility for workloads, because the allocation, monitoring and evaluation of service delivery can only be performed on the basis of knowledge of tasks to be done, demands made and individual worker strengths and weaknesses. It is a critical part of worker support and should be performed by the front line manager who could then enable the process which could be seen as *care management* at all levels.

Summary

Having undertaken an analysis and comparison of the skills, values and tasks involved in care management we have proceeded in this chapter to offer a model for the management of care management. Whether services are provided from the statutory, voluntary or independent sector, there is a need for a line management function which will support the care managers, and others carrying out functions within the care management process, in the performance of their task. The management of care management goes further than mere support, because budgetary devolution demands a new set of skills from a manager, giving that manager more control over decisions such as levels of service and sources of provision of service, all related to cost.

It is this twofold function that makes it imperative that line managers address the issue of workloads, both the measurement of workloads and their management. We maintain that a consideration of who does what, how tasks are defined and how they compare with each other is essential for the effective functioning of care management. The next section of the book therefore outlines a model of workload management related directly to the summary of care management which follows in the next chapter.

6

A Framework for Good Care Management

Introduction

Previous chapters have sought to introduce, describe and explain a number of interlocking themes which can be summarised as follows.

1. The thrust towards a still greater commitment to caring for people in the community. As a society, for three or four decades now, we have tried to tackle what has increasingly been seen as our over-dependence on residential services – large homes for children and elderly people, long-stay hospitals and, most recently prisons.
2. The view that both the process of transition to community care, as well as the task of caring for people in their own homes, or in 'homely' settings, will not lead to a better quality of social care unless it is carefully organised. A primary concern of this book is to argue that conscientious organisation and management are essential at all levels, from the overview of service plans, to the detailed delivery of services. Our particular focus is on effective management at the front line.
3. The potential for chaos, not to mention the already observable reality (like the number of ex-hospital

patients now homeless on city streets), certainly cries out for good management, but no amount of managerial talent will make up for insufficient resources. Better management cannot compensate for inadequate funding.

4. The system for coping with community care, preferred by the Conservative Government and in varying stages of development in the personal social services, is *care management*. This is a way of responding to clients, to help them identify and meet their needs, and a way of organising the assessment of needs and the provision of services. It is a comprehensive system, requiring a setting in which there is sound workload management. In the particular British context there is an additional political agenda about the diversification of service provision, with a much larger role for the independent sector.

5. Care management will have a major impact on social workers and their front line colleagues, particularly in developing the role of enabler rather than, or alongside, that of direct provider. Many of the skills and practices of care management are familiar to social workers, especially those who have experience of multi-disciplinary teamwork, linking with the voluntary and private sector, and using group or community work approaches. Some new skills are demanded, especially in resource management and balancing the claims of improved productivity with those of best professional practice.

6. A number of diverse tasks are identified in care management, including assessment, planning the care package, providing or generating the resources, contracting and arranging the provision of services, ensuring that the client's views are heard, dealing with problems and complaints, and overseeing the implementation and quality of the service the client gets. The care manager may have a wide responsibility in all of this, but will need support from others. Care management is a team activity.

7. In any workload management system the role of front line manager is vital, as allocator of tasks, monitor of overall workloads, and the person responsible for a wide range of activities which contribute to team welfare and efficiency, such as quality of work, the way emergencies and sudden surges of demand are met, and staff development. In most instances the team manager combines the roles of representative of the employer and professional supervisor. Within a care management system the front line manager may be the service manager, the person responsible for overseeing the management of all cases held by the team.

8. Care management is an activity which also requires proper regard to the views and aspirations of consumers. This consumerist characteristic in turn forces attention onto the nature of the consumer group and the society within which needs arise. It is a multi-cultural society, and one in which sensitivity and active intervention are needed to insure against discrimination.

9. There are extensive agency implications to operating a care management system. The most sensitive issue is that of devolution, of ensuring that those who are to manage cases have the necessary control over resources and decision making (as well, of course, as a sufficiency of resources). Amongst the important support services are comprehensive information, quickly and easily accessible, training, and technical expertise in such areas as contracting.

Such themes have emerged from the detailed debate in earlier chapters about the impact of modern ideas, pressures and developments on social work practices. Care management is one such development, but there are others which cannot be ignored. The formation of social services departments started the long-term process of diversifying from casework into the broader spectrum of personal social servicing. The thrust to be creative about community care, and reduce dependence on residential resources, has a still longer history, dating at least from the 1959 Mental Health Act. Years of austerity, coupled to a dominant political philosophy which draws heavily on private industry for exemplars of good practice, have put a spotlight on tighter resource management, cost-effectiveness measures, customer responsiveness and performance indicators. Social work is under pressure to change and is changing. It may have some of the qualities of art, or indeed science, but it is well on the way to becoming a business.

This chapter and the next take the analysis a stage further, first of all by seeking to draw these themes together into an overview of a flexible framework for employing care management and then by identifying how workloads will need to be properly managed in such a framework. In tackling the first of these tasks, we feel that it would be pointless to produce a single rigid structure for care management. Flexibility is vital, to encourage sensitivity to local services, to enable changes to be made in response to growing experience of these new approaches, and to acknowledge that there are differing theoretical designs for care management. Perhaps the most helpful approach at this stage is to identify the content of care management in a systematic way, and spell out the important choices that have to be made at each stage in the process.

From an agency perspective a care management system also has to sit comfortably alongside other ways of assessing and providing services. The only expectation placed on social services departments by the legislation is that they will develop care management for particular client groups. There is, as yet at least, no requirement covering all clients, and most significantly no guidance relating to child care. Some agencies may wish to reject care management altogether, or develop it as the core approach to meeting needs, rather than cope with the inconvenience of running different systems in parallel. Others will accept such differences, and so have individual social workers with a mix of clients, some of whom are handled in traditional ways and others who are 'care managed'. The variety of modes adopted has already been explored in Chapter 4. Vital features of care management, such as attitudes to devolution and the arrangement of agency information, will be sensitive to the choice each agency makes as to where care management is to sit on the spectrum between peripheral activity and central service delivery system.

The framework for care management

It has already been stated that care management is a mix of old and new, familiar and unfamiliar. In the preceding three chapters we have examined in some detail how parts will be breaking new ground, while much will remain on well-trodden territory. The fact that something is stated as a principle, a technique or a feature of care management does not imply that it is fundamentally different from the better established ways in which we seek to meet client needs. The extent of continuity will also make the model appear frequently (probably irritatingly) to experienced social workers rather like repeating the basic alphabet of their professional knowledge, skills and values, 'teaching Granny to suck eggs'.

For example, there is a sound and rarely challenged value in social work – 'start where the client is' – which provides a suitable beginning for a structure of care management. From this starting-point it is possible to construct a pathway, based partly on a chronological sequence of contacts with the client or customer, and partly on the stage in the process when particular requirements become apparent. The pathway is set out below:

1. *Client contact.* The initial presentation of need.
2. *Recording and tracking.* Starting the sequence of contacts and the data collection and recording which formally establishes the client as a customer of the agency.

3. *Assessment.* The process being introduced in the UK as a legal right of those client groups for whom care management is recommended.
4. *Advocacy.* Ensuring the strong involvement or representation of the client/customer's viewpoint.
5. *Choosing a care manager.* Identifying the person in the social services agency who is to have an overview and overall responsibility for enabling the customer/client's needs to be met.
6. *Planning the care package.* Identifying the services required to meet needs, the cost and potential location of the services, and the intended outcomes of service provision.
7. *The framework for purchasing the care package.* (a) devolution and resource flexibility – providing an administrative and support system which facilitates the execution of the role of the care manager; (b) resource raising and brokerage – identifying and generating a broad base for the resources which will be used to provide the care package.
8. *Putting the care package into action.* The service purchasing process.
9. *Providing the care package*: (a) initiating services – mobilising the chosen range of services and ensuring their provision to the client/customer; (b) maintaining the care package – establishing high quality provision, dealing with problems and complaints, and initiating reviews in the light of developments and outcome targets.
10. *Involving the independent sector.* Current and future scope to move outside the traditional UK system of direct provision through central and local government agencies.

As part of the context for this pathway some attention has to be paid to the agency (or agencies) in which the care manager and other purchasers or providers operate. Hence it is relevant to draw attention to the role of senior agency managers and especially the service manager.

1. *Client contact: start where the client is.* Care management is a development of the concept of a needs-led service and incorporates values to do with the role of consumers–customers. For that reason alone the client is the appropriate starting point, but it is also the necessary beginning for an understanding of a service delivery system.

If we start the framework with a heading 'Client Contact', then it is necessary to be able to identify who makes up the actual and potential client group. At moments of indiscretion and idealism Britain has sought to make this identification by surveying and keeping a register of all those who could come into these categories. This was the situation in the early 1970s following the Chronically Sick and Disabled Person's Act; it has for many years been the intention in the context of children at risk. In some instances, as with offenders coming before the courts, the potential client population is defined by activity elsewhere in our social system.

In practice we have tended to use less than comprehensive ways of tracing those with needs, often because of an awareness that more thorough routes would simply generate more need than the services could handle. It is standard practice for agencies to be reactive, making use of the difference between *need* and *demand*. With a few client groups, such as children at risk or placed on supervision through a court order, there is a responsibility to maintain awareness of the total population of those groups. Other clients are identified only if the need they have is brought before an agency, by a process of referral, and comes to represent a request or demand for service. It is argued, no doubt with some relevance, that the difference between the need for help and an application to a public agency is a reflection of how many needs are met through self-help, or action by friends, relatives and local networks. Nevertheless it is also well known in relation to some provisions, such as welfare benefits, that leaving it to the needy person to make an application results in a level of take-up well below the level of need. There is no reason to suppose that matters are any different across the personal social services. For all sorts of reasons, for example, lack of knowledge or ability to apply, the distance or inaccessibility of the local social services office, scepticism about the likely agency reaction, or feelings of estrangement and stigma, many people do not come forward. It is amongst the particularly deprived parts of society, and amongst minority cultures, that the ability and willingness to apply for help is lowest. Overall a reactive stance by the social services in the identification of need is scarcely likely to promote equality of opportunity.

If agencies want to be more than sensitive to need, then there are well established procedures, such as using demographic data to pinpoint vulnerable groups, or linking into sources of local knowledge (church, community centre, community activists and so forth) to unearth people's needs. What is required in the planning process is honesty, being clear whether a 'client group' indicates a level of need in the community or arises from a more restricted approach.

2. *Recording and tracking.* The data needed for care management are in part material about clients. A vital choice to be made is whether a record starts at the point where a person is formally noted as 'a referral', that is a potential client for assessment, or whether it starts at the point where a need is identified. The former equates the client information system with the agency caseload: the latter includes the caseload, but goes further afield into making a record of known needs, whether or not they lead directly to a referral. Three reasons suggest that the latter ought to be the choice. The first is political, reiterating the argument just made, that if only referrals are recorded, rather than all known need, then agency information systems will institutionalise the discrimination which arises from ignoring those whose needs do not come to agency attention.

The other two reasons have a more direct practical impact on agency functioning. One is the extent to which material about both caseloads and needs is useful in long-term planning or simply 'being prepared'. Knowledge derived from referrals and caseloads is not a sound basis for planning future services, or deciding on the allocation of staff and other resources. We know that referrals represent only a proportion of needs in a given community, and agencies cannot control the stability of such a situation. There are too many examples where plans have been thrown into disarray because some event or change in attitudes has put a spotlight on the previously shadowy group of those with needs who have never come forward for help. British social services agencies, for example, have learned by bitter experience that a passive reactive attitude towards children's needs can and has led to tragedies. Much the same happens with elderly people whenever there is particularly cold weather. Some of those who need help and do not get it are left to die.

The final reason is linked to the fact that social servicing is not a one-off event. It may be continuous, as with a person with serious physical disabilities; it may be episodic, like respite help for a carer: or it may be something which is not warranted at present, but will be at some point in the future. In all these patterns the notion of *tracking* is important, whether for tracing people through agency records, or more literally for keeping track of people with needs as their circumstances change, or as they change locality. The more comprehensive the client data kept on the information system, the easier it is to maintain effective tracking.

There is an issue here about the way gathering personal data, especially when linked to facilities for searching the data and identifying separate bits of data with the name of an individual, intrudes on personal privacy and threatens confidentiality. Information systems which serve the purposes of a comprehensive and detailed tracking of people's needs are likely to be vast, all-inclusive and computerised for easy manipulation. The notion of confidentiality has to be extremely elastic if it is to apply. A client's personal details in a file seen only by a social worker, records clerk and front line manager can be described as confidential: but can the same be said if that material is open to several hundreds or even thousands of authorised users of an agency's computer system? There is a real dilemma. On the one hand it can be argued, as we have just done, that an information system should be as broadly based as possible, linked to need in a community, not just to those who come forward to ask for, or demand, a service. This sort of information system, as stated, will tend to be huge and intrusive. On the other hand a smaller more selective information system, or even more a decision (in the interests of confidentiality) not to keep records, can lead to agencies being wholly unprepared for the challenges placed on them, unable to move in planned anticipation of real need for help. The importance of devising for social services agencies a comprehensive information system which permits proactivity to prevent damage, and is at the same time ethically acceptable, is discussed later in the chapter.

3. *Assessment.* Good assessment has always been at the heart of effective social work. Within the current debate about care management in Britain it is put under the spotlight, partly because of the view that some assessment processes have become sloppy (especially too tied in with awareness of limited service facilities) and partly because of the idea that all potential clients should have a right to be assessed by a social services department, even if they are not subsequently offered help or go to another agency for service.

It follows that an assessment should have a number of characteristics:

(a) It should be available on demand. For this reason (and others which are to do with anti-discriminatory practice) the assessment agency must be equipped to carry out assessments using a range of methods of communication (different languages and non-verbal routes) and with an understanding of a range of cultures.

(b) It should be self-contained, because it has to be potentially transferrable to another agency.

(c) It should cover the identification of needs and any formal processes for calculating eligibility, though in care management's separation of the purchaser and provider roles the assessment may not make specific servicing proposals.

(d) The assessment should be sensitive to the possibility of distortion resulting from the assessor's knowledge of currently available local services. A matter for consideration is whether there should be some degree of separation between the assessor and whoever might then take responsibility for planning services.

(e) It should reflect the views of the consumer as well as those of the professional assessor.

(f) The presentation and ownership of the assessment are important. Traditionally in most British agencies the assessment is viewed as an internal record, as part of the client file, and used as the basis for determining services and ongoing review. In the context of a more mixed economy of welfare, and where a right exists to assessment but not service, it may be appropriate to provide a separate assessment document (without excluding the role of the assessment in a more continuous record). In many, perhaps all circumstances, it may be appropriate to acknowledge consumers' right to assessment by handing a copy of the document to them, which they can take, if they wish, to other agencies.

4. *Advocacy*. The participation of the client–consumer in assessment is an integral part of social work practice, though it is acknowledged that this may not, perhaps cannot occur with people who become clients through obligation rather than choice. On the care management agenda are both the nature and the effectiveness of consumer involvement. There are circumstances in which the consumer's view of needs may differ from that of the professional assessor,

either through disagreement or interpretation. The latter is a more complex matter and is illustrated, for example, in that aspect of social work theory which distinguishes between the 'presenting problem' (that is the consumer's view of affairs) and the 'underlying situation' (the outcome of the social worker's analysis). Care management theory has ducked this kind of issue, but has pressed to ensure that the consumer's views are represented in the assessment.

The ability of consumers to state their views has been highlighted in recent debates, often drawing on an approach developed for clients with learning difficulties or physical disabilities. This is the notion of a client representative, designated as advocate, who is charged to get to know the consumer's views (not always an easy task), make sure they are effectively stated, and generally represent the consumer's position. Advocacy is part of the wider process of care management, but not a task of the care manager. Indeed the task of the advocate to represent the client's position could well lead to a need to confront and challenge the service agencies. Given such a possibility there is a strong case for the advocate being outside the agency employment structure, away from pressures to reflect agency interests.

The role of the advocate has been lodged adjacent to assessment. In the care management process this is where advocacy begins to be important, though this is also no more than a starting-point. Where there is a need for an advocate, such need is likely to continue throughout the consumer's contact with service agencies, with stages of special emphasis, such as planning the care package, overseeing the delivery of services and contributing to reviews.

Agencies have to make some choices about advocacy. They may choose to have no involvement, leaving the matter unattended or for some other initiative. They may identify the need for advocacy, perhaps as part of the assessment, but go no further. They may provide an advocacy service, despite reservations mentioned earlier. Or they may be active in helping someone else (perhaps another organisation or carer) to provide advocacy. An issue for out-of-agency advocacy is that advocates need recruiting and careful selection, which may not always be easy; they are also likely to need training and ongoing support. The possibility that advocates may operate as individuals, or from a voluntary service, should not minimise the importance of them having considerable expertise, including an ability to communicate, plan and argue with professional service providers.

    5. *Choosing a care manager.* Earlier we looked in some detail at the implications of having care managers who are not social workers. There are particular skills demanded in care management, some of which are already possessed by social workers (such as working out how needs can best be met). At the same time there are other skills not currently in the social worker's make-up; that is, until new training is provided. Despite anguish felt by many social workers, it is hard to justify their claimed monopoly of all care management roles. A sound principle might be to require a section in the assessment outlining, first of all, whether a care management approach is suitable for that particular client and, if it is, what sort of care manager would be best. In many instances a social worker will be the most suitable choice, but there are many situations where some other professional, or indeed the client, might do a better job.

    In practice it is the skills, values, philosophy and quality of the individual that are more important than the job label or the professional qualification, at least for as long as the UK has no specific training for would-be care managers. Even then there are other significant concerns. The care manager's role is one of considerable responsibility, and the ability to meet such responsibility requires not only skills, but also authority to do the job. Certainly it is necessary to appoint a care manager who is appropriate in terms of the needs of the client. At the same time that person must have a standing in the agency, and in relation to service colleagues, which facilitates the task. Generally social workers have such standing, and it is necessary to ensure that others who are appointed as care managers also have it. This includes the situation when a client is perceived as a possible care manager. We shall return to this issue later, in the context of the devolution of control of resources.

6. *Planning the care package.* At the moment when attention focuses on preparing a package of care it must be assumed that needs are known and eligibility for service has been established (both as part of the assessment). Eligibility is not always a matter of straightforward calculation, nor of clear decision. With welfare benefits there is precision – a claimant is either eligible for benefit or not. With most services there is a much more complex set of priorities for service allocation. A number of factors are taken into account. Some are client-related, as with the severity and urgency of need, and an assessment of likely trends – will the need go away if ignored, or will it get worse? Some are resource related, such as the availability of staff and other facilities. In care management the resource calculation will include the supply of money to purchase services. Statutory obligation also plays a part, giving a higher rating to someone whose needs are covered by law. The prospect of a successful outcome is a further factor, and one that will become more important as techniques of cost–benefit analysis are developed.

The task under care management is to take into account the amount of resource that is required, but not to be circumscribed either by knowledge of specific services available for direct provision or even by a knowledge of existing provisions in the locality. There are two theoretical principles here (some might prefer to view them as ideals): that services must fit client needs, not vice versa, and that services can be created to match needs. Within this dual focus the planned care package is a statement of the services recommended for the client, and the resources available to obtain them. The desired services will be accompanied by a justification of how they derive from the assessment, what their provision is expected to achieve, over what period, and what goals should be set and reviewed. Indication of the client's understanding and agreement is also important.

The part of the package relating to resources presents choices. In its purest mixed economy version it will be a declaration of the sum allocated to purchase services, perhaps accompanied by a statement of the client's contribution, funds from other sources and plans to raise money or services. In this context services will be purchased from a market which includes in-agency facilities as well as the independent sector. In a less radical format the statement may well seek to distinguish at this stage between services for direct provision, and plans to make purchases externally. Some agencies may well seek to minimise the move away from direct service provision, and their success will depend on the political climate.

The 'services' which have been referred to are wide ranging. They include all the existing in-house provisions, such as residential and day care facilities, home care and, most vitally for social workers, their own time as counsellors, therapists, group workers, or whichever of their skills are needed. Externally they include all those services and aids already provided by, for example, voluntary groups and the National Health Service. Additionally it is hoped that the focus on planning to meet people's needs in a flexible environment will lead to imaginative new types of service. Last but not least, care management itself, this new enabling role for social workers and others, joins the list.

7. *The framework for purchasing the care package.* Within the British setting the development of care management has been closely linked to the (politically determined) target of moving away from direct service provision by public service agencies, mainly social services departments, towards a mixed arrangement of public and private agencies. Part of the process of putting this aim into operation is the identification of assessment as a distinct and separate task, so allowing clients to have their needs established quite in-

dependently of any tendency to match them, from the start, to known services. A further operational approach had been the distinction drawn between *purchaser* and *provider* roles. The social services department is the purchaser of services: more specifically the care manager is the purchaser, for each client, of the agreed care package, within the limit of available resources. In the vast majority of cases, at least into the foreseeable future, the social services department will also be the sole or major provider of services, whether through political commitment or through the pragmatic acknowledgement that at the moment, in many areas of service provision, there are no other agencies around to do the job.

It follows that social services departments have some important issues to decide in relation to their role in the market as both purchaser and provider. There is a spectrum of opportunity, in theory at least. At one end of the spectrum the agency develops the notion of an internal market, and structures itself with a clear division between those with purchaser and those with provider responsibilities. On the purchasing side is the assessor, the care manager and supports such as tendering, quality control and complaints units. On the providing side are all those directly involved in the face-to-face task of offering help to clients. At the other end of the spectrum is a much more confused position in which many staff, including care managers, carry out purchasing and providing tasks, often using long-established practices, and commonly with little awareness of purchaser–provider divisions.

In reality the crisply divided internal market may be hard to achieve. Some resources are not so conveniently divisible or, if enforced would open up the sorts of demarcation issues which were recorded as the bane of British industry in the 1970s. At one end of the hierarchy centralised planning and management would be challenged, while at the front line staff could face seriously disruptive role confusion. Nevertheless just to ignore the division makes it much harder for a client to obtain an assessment which is a genuine reflection of need, and not contaminated by the assessor's knowledge of the availability (or, more significantly, non-availability) of particular services. It is also harder to negotiate a care package and make a clear identification of the resources which can be allocated, as well as to be more open to the independent sector.

Somewhere within the spectrum there has to be a working compromise, which, as already stated with as much firmness as we can muster, will be much easier to achieve if adequate resources are provided. For the present, some attention can be given to two aspects of the purchasing arrangement, 'flexing' and raising resources.

(a) *Devolution and resource flexibility*. The moment resource matters come to the forefront in care management, the model has to take account of the two issues of devolution and flexibility. Both affect agency management practices as a whole. The former raises the issue of devolving control over budgeting to the level in the hierarchy of service or care management. Choices include devolution right down to the care manager, or less fragmentation of budgetary decisions by giving the service manager a pivotal role. Other options, as already mentioned, are influenced by the central or peripheral place of care management in agency service provision.

Resource flexibility concerns the intention of matching provisions to client needs. A flexible resource is something which is responsive to requests to change, for example to change location or function. The most flexible resource is money; but though money may be used in many ways, converting it into a required service (think of using it to train another social worker, or any occupational therapist) can take an unacceptably long time. A more realistic option is to put into the model consideration of: (i) increasing the flexibility of existing provisions by assessing the extent to which they can be freed from restrictive rules, regulations and practices regarding their use (an example would be scope to vire between different budget categories in response to changes in demand); (ii) developing information sources and analysis which allow frequent detailed projections of changes in types of service provision being requested in care packages; and (iii) giving a high priority in service development to the establishment of multi-purpose resources, including staffing; integral to the staffing aspect of such an option is a proactive training facility, and perhaps a corps of mobile staff. In theory, though not so attractive in practice, flexibility can be increased by (iv) maintaining surplus capacity, such as spare places in day centres or respite care, to meet new demands. An analogy here is with the idea of a shop keeping stocks of a commodity, in preparation for a paying customer. Should agencies keeps stocks of service resources, so as to be able to respond to a wish to purchase?

(b) *Resource raising and brokerage.* One of the Conservative Government's aspirations in promoting care management was that it would incorporate actions to increase the resources available to the personal social services. This notion of resource generation can be viewed at different levels in the agency hierarchy, or even as a wider (for example, local government) activity. At the level of the agency, linkages to major foundations the establishment of foundations, or industrial sponsorships are all on the agenda.

The broker is another potential member of the care management team, and may not be involved solely in resource generation. Resource generation covers many activities, from raising money to mobilising and helping local communities to develop a helping role. It can be an activity directly linked to helping a named client. In this form the resource raiser or broker may be a local volunteer or someone in the client's immediate circle, such as a relative or friend, and may also be involved in tasks such as advocacy. Another model views the broker more as a professional fund raiser or community organiser working from the local social services office on behalf of many clients on the caseload.

8. *Putting the care package into action.* Once the desired package of care is known, and decisions made about

resources to be allocated, the task is then to obtain the best services possible within the resource ceiling. In addressing the agenda and options for this part of the care management model it might be helpful to begin with the approach which is nearest to the free market, and then look at the more familiar scene in which the social services department is the main service provider.

The free market approach immediately calls attention to three themes and one issue surrounding the service purchasing activity:

(a) Tendering. The care manager is expected to seek services which offer best value for money and involve a professional judgement about the balance of quality with cost. A route to this is competitive tendering, through which potential service providers are invited to state their costs for a given service. This tender and any subsequent contract may relate to a service for a specific client, or to a block of services for a number of clients. All of the processes involved, drawing up an invitation to tender, submitting a tender, and assessing the quality of a tender, are known from experience elsewhere in the economy to be complex and skilled tasks, requiring specialised ability. The care manager will need special training or skilled help to handle the purchasing side, and will also need to be sure that the person or organisation submitting a tender is competent at the task.

(b) Services are then contracted by the purchaser from a provider. Again there are tasks of drawing up and negotiating contracts which require skills on both sides. The system cannot assume that only the purchaser (care management) side is skilled at this task, because incompetence on the provider side can lead (already has led!) lead to contracts failing, and the client suffering. As with tendering, specialist help and training are essential.

(c) In order to purchase services the care manager (or whoever is doing the buying) needs extensive information, on the availability of service suppliers, the features of their services, the quality of offerings from the different suppliers and prices. In the commercial sector of the economy there is a massive body of information in catalogues, databases, the files of experienced operatives and known reputations. Little of this kind is currently available in social services departments, so it will need to be built up quite quickly. The development of approved lists of service providers is a first step towards this database. As with the earlier reference to client data, this is another of the new information needs if care management is to be successful.

The core issue surrounding this whole aspect of the care management process is that of the relationship between purchaser and provider. Keeping to a radical line, one feature of the system might well be a substantial separation between those roles, so that a market-led relationship can exist unencumbered by other links. By that is meant a relationship in which the tendering, contracting and subsequent service evaluation processes are not impeded. This would apply even where the service provider was part of the same agency. Indeed, as we have acknowledged, a typical system could well be that the care manager purchased services primarily from within that person's own locality and own agency. The alternative route is based on the argument that, since for the majority of transactions the purchaser and provider are part of the same agency, in all probability the same team, such a formal division of roles is pointless and contrary to best agency practice.

This brings us onto more familiar territory, where putting the care plan into action involves a mixture of seeking resources through traditional channels from within the agency and filling out the package, perhaps also through traditional channels, by going to other agencies or looking for volunteers.

The traditional channels which social workers use within social services departments include making a case for a client to an allocation panel, applying through the hierarchy for a particular resource, or simply allocating some of their own time to helping the client. The criterion for success is not purchasing power, but establishing the priority claim of that particular client.

Depending on how the care package is set up, the notions of purchasing and cash values may or may not have a place. If the care plan does state resource allocations in terms of cash, then the service allocations may be expressed in the form of their cash cost, as a paper transaction. If the care package lists resources simply in the form of services to be allocated, then cash values may be totally absent. However an important feature to remember about care management, one which is different from most traditional practices, is the stress placed on the care manager knowing the cost of the services being provided, and being able to make both assessments of value for money, and comparisons with packages for other clients.

9. *Providing the care package.* It was said of the activities which led to the merger of many small agencies into large social services departments in 1971 – and it is being said again of current moves towards community care, care management and the development of a mixed economy of welfare – that all the preoccupation is with administrative matters. New structures, systems and procedures are being debated and mulled over, with the tendency to forget that what is important in the last resort is that people get good quality services which meet their needs, and the staff to provide those services.

However there are short- and long-term dimensions to the task of service provision, initiating the services agreed in the care package, and then maintaining them through their allotted time and intensity, it is hoped until they have achieved their objectives.

(a) *Initiating and commissioning services.* One of the

criticisms of large hierarchical organisations (as many social services departments are held to be) is that they take good staff away from direct work with clients into the nether regions of administration. Often the criticism is unwarranted. Good staff are needed for developmental work, or to keep a steady hand on the agency tiller, as well as to provide services. Nevertheless it is an observation with some truth in it that agency restructuring often takes experienced people away from the front line, leaving less experienced staff to do the job. A system which draws care managers back from direct service provision could have the same impact, putting great emphasis on their role as initiators, enablers and supporters of services.

There are a number of specific tasks for the care manager once the care package has been formulated, resources established and providers identified. Introductions have to be made and relationships formed with the client and significant people in the client's network, such as a carer or advocate. If there are several providers then there is an immediate task of co-ordination and a longer-term task of team-building. Job divisions need to be clarified, the different professional inputs marked up, and early activities monitored to ensure that what was planned is actually happening. If there is an administrative point to make, it is that the care manager's task has only just begun when the care package is purchased. It has to be made to work.

(b) *Maintaining the care package.* The care manager may or may not be part of the service provider network for a given client, but s/he will have responsibility for monitoring the progress of the care package, keeping the client's needs and their fit with service provisions under review, and deciding at what point service should stop, or a process of reassessment be undertaken. This is not the only level of review and monitoring. Consumers will be involved, as will service providers themselves. Input therefore occurs at a number of levels. Two aspects in particular are likely to be aided by central developments within each social services department: (i) there should be a procedure already in place to deal with complaints or suggestions about any particular aspect of community care; and (ii) most departments are seeing a central responsibility for overall quality assurance, though the targets for quality assurance activities vary. At one end of the scale they may be confined to specified in-house services. At the other end they may range widely across in-house services, including the quality of care management, and extend into quality checks on independent sector provisions. Suitable methods for assessing service quality, especially in the independent sector, are in their infancy, though a clear role is emerging for evaluations based on the views of consumers. Another variation in the model is that many departments appear to be choosing to link quality assurance with formal inspectoral functions.

10. *The independent sector.* The free market model of service purchasing tends to assume a kind of independent sector which may develop in the future, but does not exist at present. It is a picture of the social services department, or the care manager, relating to and forming contracts with a range of business-like organisations. They differ from other manufacturing and commercial companies in that their output is services, and they may be non-profit companies, but they are seen as functioning through market procedures for getting and meeting contracts.

Because this is not a picture of current reality, social services departments, as purchasing agencies, will have to play an active role in creating such an independent sector over quite a long transitional phase. Help will have to be given to set up appropriate forms of administration; training may have to be provided; perhaps even some investment will have to be made to stimulate independent activity. In practice a few local authorities have aided the process by allowing or encouraging social services staff to operate what amounts to a management buy-out of limited services, like the provision of residential care, but this has not been on the basis of competitive tendering. The allocation of the contract to a private security firm for electronic tagging indicates the possibilities in the penal field and the 'sponsoring' of nurses by drug companies is a development in the health field. A model of working with the independent sector which focuses on that sector as it is at present has to accept a number of limitations. There is what can be called 'businesslike' organisation and behaviour in relatively small pockets of activity, most significantly in private residential care. Within the context of community care the independent sector consists predominantly of a range of voluntary and non-profit groups. Some are national organisations with local branches, like the Women's Royal Voluntary Service (WRVS) and the Red Cross. Others are small and locally based. Despite having some salaried staff, almost all depend on volunteers as the main labour force, and by their nature voluntary workers are keen, but often unable to match professional expectations of skill or reliability. Few community care groups in the independent sector would be both available to sell services and dependable enough to make a contract with.

In such a context a temptation will be for the care manager to identify the priority elements of the care package and place them either for direct provision or with the small number of suitable agencies elsewhere (including other social services departments). Only relatively low priority parts of the package could find their way into the independent sector. However, if there is to be commitment to the principle of an independent sector (which, of course, is a political decision), then effective practice will only develop if there is a determined and patient attempt to stimulate the independent market.

According to the type of system in use and the purchaser–provider structure, the care management system will include elements of vetting contracts to check that they are being observed, coping with broken or unsatisfactory contracts, and book-keeping to ensure that resource allocations are not being overspent. There can also be tasks linked to the existence and continuing role of support staff, such as advocates and brokers. As argued earlier, care management is a team activity and, like any team, it will need support as well as opportunities to reflect and develop.

Central services

Many of these have been mentioned in the process of following through the pathway of the care management process. However, by way of summarising, it is pertinent to point out that senior agency managers have a role in enabling the successful implementation of care management. Policies towards devolution and resource flexibility have been mentioned. Support is implied for new roles, for example in advocacy and brokerage. There are major training and personnel implications to be worked out. A system of workload management has to be put in place and supported, to offer a framework within which care management can be productive. Technical help is needed in matters like tendering and contracting, which may most easily be handled through a centrally based specialised team. Complaints and quality assurance procedures need to function in a way which enhances rather than undermines the work of front line staff. Departmental care plans must be developed. Substantial information needs have to be acknowledged. Perhaps most of all, adequate resources have to be found. Although most of the above have been discussed already one central service which has been alluded to consistently is the provision of an appropriate infrastructure for gathering, processing and disseminating information.

Information needs

Looking back over the characteristics of care managing community care services, we can begin to identify the sorts of information required, a large part of which seems likely to be computer based. The dominant themes are those of (1) range of information, (2) presentation of information, (3) devolution of information, (4) information for consumers and (5) information and best practice.

Range of information. Existing information systems tend to contain client files, and material about directly provided services. There are two main areas of expansion needed for care management:

(a) financial information and budgetary systems, not only of the sort used in overall planning, but linked to devolved budgets, and to care package costs for individual clients; and

(b) information about the independent sector, its resources, capacities, skills, charges, and so forth.

Presentation of information. In the context of workload management at the level of the individual case and/or locality or client group caseloads, effective care management depends on substantial information sources and databases. Data are needed in relation to clients, services and budgets.

Client information is needed which:

(a) stores needs assessments for client (and their representative, advocate or carer);

(b) stores (or helps make) recommendations on care packages, including priority rating in relation to client needs and (means tested) eligibility;

(c) states the budget allocated to client with full details of expenditure on that budget; and

(d) Copies the care package contract, specifying what will be provided directly, what will be purchased with allocated resources, what other agencies will be pressed to provide at their expense, what resource raising will be supported for the client, and what is not to be pursued.

Service information covers:

(a)   availability of specific services, with particulars of source, cost, delivery time, quality rating, referees/references, informed persons, contracting/purchasing arrangements, special conditions (such as minimum purchase) and so forth; this amounts to an on-line catalogue which care manager and client can draw on in preparing to implement a care package, and fitting desired services to the budget available;

(b)   scope for the care manager and client to ask 'If . . .' questions about potential care packages (for example, 'If we needed transport on three afternoons each week, who could provide it, and what would it cost?'); and for agency managers to be able to understand the wider and longer-term impact on staff and other facilities of care package decisions; and

(c)   resource files on voluntary agencies, charities and so on. Also, relevant, a directory of volunteers, with information about their skills, availability, linked costs, quality rating and so on.

Budgetary material covers:

(a)   client means testing, service costs and an on-line accountancy facility linked to running totals of the cost implications of care packages agreed for implementation;

(b)   administration of generated income (cash and kind); and

(c)   if appropriate, administration of a voucher or token system.

Devolution of information.   The framework for the devolution of access to information systems arises from whatever decisions are taken about the devolution of budgetary and decision-making responsibilities for community care by social services departments. *Caring for People* is not prescriptive on this matter, but (para.3.3.5) 'the Government sees advantage in linking care management with delegated responsibility for budgetary management. This need not be pursued down to the level of each individual client in all cases, but – used flexibly – is an important way of enabling those closest to the identification of client needs to make the best possible use of the resources available.' This statement suggests that the degree/level of devolution should be variable, but in some instances will be down to the level of individual cases. Whatever happens in relation to particular cases, the system should be flexible. It follows that access to the information necessary for the effective implementation of such delegation will also have to be flexible.

This sort of flexibility will, in the first instance, depend on the deployment of equipment offering access to the agency's information systems. In some social services departments this has already occurred down to area office or other major service location (like a large hospital): in others such infrastructure is not in place. Even where there is a solid devolved infrastructure of information technology (IT) hardware, questions will have to be asked about usage. A widespread experience in locations like area offices is that IT equipment is mainly, sometimes wholly, used by clerical and administrative staff. Professional staff, whether from choice or lack of opportunity, often do not sit at the computer keyboard. For the majority of current uses this situation may not reflect the most helpful response to the provision of IT services, but it appears to be functional. Can the same be said of care management? Will care managers be able to work via clerical staff, and keep the computer at arm's length, or will it be essential for the care manager to have, on his or her desk, the means of access to essential information? By simply posing such questions it is difficult to escape the conclusion that care managers will have to be provided with complex hardware and software, and there will have to be corresponding changes in attitudes towards the direct use of IT by professional staff.

As well as a capital need, devolution and flexibility touch on some of the issues of the presentation of information which have already been noted. Care managers are likely to want to be able to analyse information from a variety of groups, some local authority-wide, others more closely linked to the immediate service locality. For example, there may be cost differences between localities, linked to such factors as travel time for home visits or charges made by independent local groups.

Information for consumers.   Two external groups are significant here, clients and sub-contractors. The process which takes place between client and care manager, possibly involving others, such as the client's carer or advocate, starts with an assessment of needs leading to the preparation of a care package to meet those needs. At this point, or concurrently with the task of designing the individualised care package, resource questions have to be asked and answered. On the basis of the assessment of the client, what is the priority to be given to the identified needs? What budget will be allocated in order to pay for the package? This in turn leads to negotiation about the package which is to be implemented, and decisions about what is direct provision, what will be sought elsewhere, and what may be desirable but is as yet unresourced. A broker or fund/resource raiser may join in for this sequence.

The issue for the information system is what material will be provided in this context for client, carer, advocate or broker? *Caring for People* takes a much diluted consumerist view, concerned solely with the facts about services which are to be offered. A firmer consumerist approach might argue that in the negotiation of packages the client side should have the same access to information as the care manager, which means not just being given selected facts, but being able to interrogate the system (including on such matters as quality and cost assessment of services), and having space to enter the client viewpoint. If community care is to do with partnership, surely this is what partnership involves? The position of sub-contractors is somewhat different. The relationship between them and the social services department is likely to be complex and, at times, confused. Many, such as voluntary organisations, have long-standing partnerships with social services at a professional level. Under the proposed new system they will interweave into this partnership the business relationship of purchaser (the care manager, inviting tenders for services) and provider (the voluntary or private group, submitting tenders and providing services).

Partnership in assisting a client requires a full sharing of information: but the business relationship also involves both sides in limiting the transfer of information to what they see as useful to their position. A voluntary organisation will discuss its weaknesses with a professional in the context of seeking to improve services, but will it do so in the context of tendering for business? At this point information, and information exchange, become a sensitive commercial matter.

Inevitably there will have to be compromise, so that a new business relationship can be established, without losing the tradition of professional trust and confidence which in itself will be vital to successful quality assurance. IT staff will be part of this process, because they will be looked to for information systems which facilitate a compromise, by allowing flexible and carefully calculated information to be produced to suit the immediate context. As an aside, it is worth noting that there is a fortune to be made by whoever produces a user-friendly, easy to operate, malleable, giving and forgiving system!

Information and best practice. The initial, and probably inevitable response to *Caring for People* (Department of Health, 1989) will be for the development of systems which aid care managers, but do so exclusively in terms of resource management. That is to say, they will focus on the supply of resources, conditions of availability, the specifics of contracts, and costs. They may, though this is dependent on data which are probably only available in agencies with existing workload management systems, go further into cost/ resource comparisons of different approaches to client needs.

The challenge for information staff, in turning a mediocre system into a first class one, will be to draw into data analysis two additional themes, service quality and professional values. First impressions are that some system designers are keen to take up this challenge. Two International Computer Limited (ICL) staff, for example (John Morris and Fraser McCluskey), have produced an internal document which sets out the principles or preconditions for a successful resource management system, one of which is 'constructive involvement of care professionals in the (choice making) managerial process'. They go on to outline the sorts of systems which will be needed in the Health and Social Services, specifying three for social services departments. One enables the interactive control of price, quantity and quality: the second is a neutral data source: the third seeks to support service delivery 'of a multi-agency care package based on multiple assessments of clients' needs'. In the last resort, of course, the choice between a narrow resource-led arrangement and one which incorporates quality, values and consumerism will depend as ever on whether the system is properly resourced.

Service management

Finally, in this overview of the concepts and processes in care management, it is important to summarise the notion of service management. Though their role in service planning should not be ignored, service managers have been defined as acting in two main areas, overseeing care management and supervising care managers. Social services departments front line community care units are traditionally organised into area centres and more specialised groups such as hospital teams. A conventional model will see care management located in these area centres (or localities), whether their internal organisation consists of specialist or generic teams. We have viewed the service manager as being in the same location, as a member of the senior staff of the area, perhaps an area manager or assistant, perhaps a team leader. In this setting the service manager will have, in many aspects, a front line management role consisting of a responsibility to maintain an overview of client needs in the area, of the service workload for the area or team, and of the performance, development and welfare of the team. Within that framework staff are both managed and offered professional supervision, and a workload management system operates.

All these continue as features of the service management role. What is added depends to a degree on decisions made about the extent of devolution, in other words about what is delegated right down to the care manager and what is kept at a more corporate and senior level. Control over area budget allocations for care packages is one possible service management task. Supervisory responsibility for advocates and brokers is also a possibility, along with the role of liaising with headquarters over centrally provided supports (like technical or legal help with contracts). If rather tentative language is being used it is because there is much flexibility in the model.

The job of supervising care managers is not intrinsically different from other professional staff supervision. Its techniques and objectives would be the same, excepting the integral role of a structured workload management system. The additional demands it would make are closely related to the job description employed for the care managers (especially when care managers who do not hold social work qualifications, or use their approaches to work, are employed). Where the care management task requires new skills and activities, for example in contracting with service providers, the service manager will need to parallel them in order to achieve effective supervision.

What is clear is that any model will need to acknowledge the workload demands of care and service management. The workload will be higher because the required tasks are more varied and intensive, demanding more skills; because more is being offered to clients (such as the comprehensive assessment); because the context is not ready-made and has to be developed (such as procedures for budgetary devolution, or working with the independent sector); because necessary information is not yet easily available; overall, because agencies will have to build up, painstakingly, the corporate experience which eventually enables any new system to work smoothly and enhances the performance of all who operate within the system.

7

Workload Management and Care Management

The workload management context

Care management is a staff intensive process, both because it represents an attempt to offer a more thoroughly prepared service to clients and because of the extra task of drawing in and co-ordinating the independent sector. From the consumer viewpoint, advocacy may also create heavy demands and the task of finding advocates may well fall to the care manager. Perhaps the greatest demand comes from the staff intensity of care management and the possibility that this will not be appreciated. If care managers are expected to handle client loads comparable to those of, say, an area team social worker, then the task could get out of hand. On the other hand, some may feel a real threat posed by the impact of devolution. If budgetary and care management powers are placed firmly in the service front line, so will big responsibilities. There can be little doubt, given the shortage of resources and the scope of the care management task, that the job of care manager will be demanding and stressful, adding to an already stressful work setting (NALGO, 1989). Careful attention will have to be paid to the content of the task, to the welfare of staff undertaking it, to their terms of service and to their training.

An argument throughout this book has been that care management can only succeed in a framework offered by a system of workload management. Traditionally the use of workload management in social work practice has been viewed as optional, often supported more in prospect than reality. Obviously there have always been managerial aspects to handling a workload, if only to provide a minimally systematic approach to keeping records, ensuring a programme of client contacts and arranging the daily diary. But many social workers have been reluctant to allow a tighter monitoring of their activities, arguing that their profession needs freedom and flexibility if their clients are to be well served. Team leaders have been obliged to use more managerial tools, especially to tackle tasks such as the fair distribution of work amongst the team, and providing sporadic reports to headquarters.

A range of factors, all of which have appeared at earlier points in this book, have increased the pressure for more managerial intervention, or more structured self-management. They are mostly connected with the trend towards increasing the volume of work placed on both social services and probation departments, but also arise in relation to the level of resources, and the growing proportion of that work is situated in a statutory setting. Legal responsibilities promote tighter systems for accountability. Increased needs command more sensitive and substantial rationing procedures. The imbalance of needs and resources puts emphasis on the use of more productive forms of service provision. There are many more such pointers, all moving social work in the direction of a more managed service. Moreover such concerns, for rationing systems, care reviews and the like, are themselves time consuming, a part of the workload: this is an observation which has hardened some attitudes against more extensive workload management.

Essentially the introduction of a care management system, in whatever form, involves introducing a front line management system. Modelling such a system for the personal social services is not simply an academic exercise: there are practical ground rules and guidelines which need to determine the process and principles from the start to avoid serious troubles at a later stage. In an earlier work (Glastonbury, Bradley and Orme, 1987) the authors set out some guidelines for implementing workload management which are worth summarising here, because the introduction of a new system to an agency, whether an overall administrative restructuring or a changed framework for service delivery, has to make best use of the available resources.

Guidelines for a front line management system

The agency's staff are its most important resource, and the largest group of guidelines were about the way staff are treated within their agencies. For instance: make sure the management system is fully understood and accepted by the front line staff who are to use it; ensure that it incorporates work allocation in a form which can enable fair and realistic workloads to be set; press staff to join in setting task measurements and weightings; use a scheme of rationing and allocation which is systematic, based on explicit priority grading, and protects coal face staff from some of the dirty jobs; keep space for staff reflection, training and development; the system needs to be sensitive to the balance of professional autonomy and accountability, and not overmanaged; participating staff need frequent feedback. Operating a workload management system as an isolated worker has particular difficulties and needs strong support.

Some guidelines offer help to front line managers. For example: keep space in work allocation for unpredictable demands; build in system reviews, with a commitment to make changes in the light of experience; be willing to take notice of all work, not just work with clients; the system needs to be sensitive to intangible staff feelings of being overworked or overstressed, and allow for such feelings, as well as more straightforward measurements, in work allocation.

Guides for more senior staff included the following: encourage system design to suit local circumstances and, conversely, do not insist on agency standardisation; within the context of encouraging locally based systems, ensure that senior staff cannot then override the system to suit a transitory purpose; do not activate a front line management system in tandem with more widespread agency restructuring, because it would involve too much change at one time; accept that there is no absolute measure of the social work task, and precision cannot be expected; do not condemn a system for initial fallibility because accuracy will improve with time; keep in mind that the personal social services are characterised by unpredictability, and this is the unavoidable back-cloth for any management system; the role of the team manager is stressful, and also needs supporting.

Just as a consistent theme in the introduction of care management is the importance of flexibility, for the same sorts of reasons there needs to be flexibility in the introduction of workload management schemes. To see workload management as a reaction to pressures, a way of squeezing more out of already harassed social workers, is to misunderstand the intentions of a proper system. Conceptually there are two parameters to a workload management system, measuring the workload of the individual or team and measuring the capacity of the resources, primarily the staff, to tackle that workload. Within those parameters the core task of a workload management system is to bring needs and resources into alignment. It is a matter of established record that needs have always exceeded resources, so the tools for securing alignment include filtering and setting priorities for needs, and subjecting them to rationing. On the supply side there must be a focus on cost-efficiency, as well as a search for methods of service provision which are productive in terms of their costs and the quantity and quality of their achievements.

Certainly these tools for coping with high levels of need are familiar to social workers, and operate outside a formal workload management system. But too often in these circumstances they operate as unregulated pressures, putting staff under stress, because they are not based on the essentials of measured needs and measured workloads. Few agencies use anything more than a rule of thumb approach in estimating the scale of the task in meeting a given need, though it has to be accepted that more sophisticated measurements do present a difficult challenge. Yet the much easier job of measuring a person's workload is also widely shirked: a recent study (NALGO, 1989) showed that only 43 per cent of a sample of 177 social workers were part of such activity. Without measurement there can be no accuracy: without accuracy there can be no clearly identified workload ceiling for staff; without a protected ceiling the pressure of needs is transferred directly to front line staff with consequent impacts on stress, capacity to cope and morale. Workload management is a system designed to make best use of staff and other resources; but it is also a system to protect staff from exploitation.

There are other benefits from the output of a workload management system. The process of measurement enhances the ease with which the state of needs and resources can be communicated, whether to senior managers or to those who make political decisions. Those same measurements are also valuable planning tools in relation to future staffing levels, and the appropriate focus of staff development and training. As we shall see, in the context of care management such measurements become essential to the whole process of care packaging and delivery.

Workload measurement and care management

In Chapter 4 we undertook a comprehensive breakdown of the tasks involved in the process of care management. It is essential for a workload management system that from the outset issues of what is to be done, by whom, and in what organisational context, are clarified in the planning stages. This is true of any changes in social work organisation and practice, and is necessary to make sure that appropriate systems are in operation to ensure that front line social workers have enough time and professional space to enable them to perform the tasks to the best of their professional ability. This requirement is not just related to the individual need for job satisfaction but is also of paramount importance when considering consumer satisfaction, quality assurance and, in care management, realistic costing.

The first concern in measuring workloads in care management is that it needs to be established that we are not just talking about the *cases* involved in care management schemes: 'Numbers alone may not prove to be a sensible way of making comparisons since the range of tasks undertaken varies so widely from project to project . . . Care in the community schemes are probably far more complex exercises than any of the case [*sic*] management schemes which have been described in other places' (Renshaw, 1988, p. 101). This complexity acknowledges that there are specific tasks within care management that can be separated and allocated. These tasks have been associated with the processes of identifying need, preparing assessments, securing services, assuring quality and reviewing. Each of these tasks has its own work implications.

For example, in the task of *identifying need* the work that needs to be done involves three stages. The first is to establish a system for making information available for potential consumers. The production and dissemination of the information in itself should be a relatively straightforward process, but a second stage involves the setting up of systems for interdisciplinary consultation. Such consultation has the potential to be stressful and time consuming. The third aspect of the process is the need to establish a system of filtering, to identify those who at that time are not in need or who do not fall into the categories for whom the agency is responsible. These cases may be more demanding than those who are referred on for detailed assessment, in that reasons will have to be given, acknowledging that the door needs to be kept open to enable them to return. Also information about other potential sources of help will need to be given. This particular analysis highlights the fact that one set of tasks vital to the care management process might not necessarily involve direct work with individual cases and would not, therefore, be counted in any notion of caseload. Even though the tasks may involve the worker in dealing with customers, these may never be counted on the agency caseload. A similar situation could arise with the function of brokerage. The broker need not have a caseload as such; the workload would require a set of identified work tasks such as attending liaison meetings, visiting existing provision and assessing it. These tasks would need monitoring and measuring so that ultimately the overall workloads of workers with different functions could be equated.

The acknowledgment that, in care management, workloads need to subsume a whole variety of activities and tasks is fundamental. Therefore there needs to be some equitable measure of what such tasks involve and the appropriate allocation to enable workers to perform them effectively. Challis and Davies (1989), for example, consistently refer to the smaller caseloads of the community care team which enabled them to perform thorough assessments. The argument that some tasks are more demanding and require more worker time and attention suggests that they should be allocated a higher weighting, whether that weighting be hours, points or any other unit. This is important because it hinges on a clear understanding of what is involved in the task and what is to be counted as 'demanding'.

In this context it is useful to consider the task of *preparing assessments* and to look at the implications of this task in determining appropriate weightings. It is a significant piece of work in its own right and therefore produces its own demands. The 'thoroughness' referred to by Challis and Davies will involve professional skills and knowledge which draw upon current social work practice, but will have to be informed by other skills and knowledge bases, such as financial management, critical awareness of the service provision available from other agencies and predictive skills to do with the longer term coping capacity of individuals. A further consideration is the scrutiny to which the assessment will be subjected. In the first instance the assessment will need to be agreed with the consumer and be seen to be meeting the identified needs. It will also have to stand up to the scrutiny of the line manager whose responsibility it is to ensure that the package which is subsequently produced on the basis of the assessment not only meets needs, but achieves the necessary support for the individual in the community and will be cost-effective. The final scrutiny will of course come from the service provider who has to implement the recommendations of the assessment. When services could be provided by a professional from a number of possible disciplines, a representative of a voluntary agency, a volunteer, an informal care or the consumers themselves, then the assessment may be subjected to wide scrutiny. The significance of this for the work involved in the assessment task therefore is that it has to be performed to an extremely high professional standard, but be accessible to all the identified consumer groups. Information to satisfy all of these demands will need to be collected in a relatively short time in order for the process of locating the services and formulating the package of care to commence and the consumer needs to be met.

Writing a comprehensive assessment for a particular purpose within given time limits (Department of Health, 1990) is not a simple task, but in the social work context it is not a totally new one. The process of writing a social inquiry report in the probation service has been identified as a discrete piece of work which meets many of the criteria outlined above. Policy initiatives within the criminal justice system (Home Office, 1990) indicate that in future this task will also involve cost-effectiveness aspects of recommendations and the identification of provisions within a mixed economy of service. What is significant for our purposes is that in the workload measurement systems of the probation service (NAPO, 1979) it is the task of writing social inquiry reports which is given the greatest time weighting. This is an acknowledgement of the actual time spent on the task which is related to the component parts of preparing an effective assessment for the purpose of the court. It is argued elsewhere (Glastonbury, Bradley and Orme, 1987) that this weighting does not necessarily reflect the stress which is involved in such a significant decision-making task. There are many parallel stresses in assessment for care management, including decisions about an individual's future; meeting deadlines; responding to the request for assessment of those in hospital beds, but under pressure to leave; and managing this demand against the ongoing assessments of those within the community who under the legislation will have the right to an assessment.

In our detail of the assessment task in Chapter 4 we suggested that the production of three assessment documents might provide the most effective outcome of the process for all the relevant groups. These 'outcomes' of the assessment process raise significant workload issues. An analysis of the task of preparing a social inquiry report revealed that probation officers spent the majority of the time preparing the written document (Orme, 1991). To suggest the completion of three documents has major implications for worker time. Similarly the suggestion that the production of an assessment can in itself be a therapeutic intervention and, in some cases, may not have a specified time period needs to be acknowledged in the workload of those involved in making the assessment.

In identifying the stresses of assessment (Chapter 4) we acknowledged that the assessments of those in hospital might take precedence over other assessments. The need for such assessments on demand highlights the unpredictability involved in identifying, measuring and balancing workloads in care management. To assume that making an assessment will only be a matter of gathering information is to deny the complexity of situations which will have to be assessed. In the past in social work practice there has been much debate about 'Part III assessments' (that is, the assessment undertaken under Part III of the 1948 National Assistance Act to establish whether an elderly person is in need of residential care). Such assessments were often seen as low-priority and used for students to 'practise' or given to unqualified workers. What is apparent is that no situation which is brought to the attention of a social worker can be assumed to be straightforward, and the cases in which assessments are being made for the purposes of care management, by virtue of the fact that they are dealing with individuals who either have chronic conditions which are liable to deteriorate, or are in acute need, are likely to be even less predictable in terms of the length and frequency of contact needed to make an appropriate and effective assessment.

This nature of the care management process, and the client group whose needs are being met by it, has further implications for unpredictability in workload terms. It will be part of a care manager's task to monitor cases for whom s/he has a responsibility and to implement *reviews*. Periodic review can comprise routine information gathering, either as a form filling exercise or as a panel discussion involving consumer, carer and any others involved. While this will involve a rise in work it is possible to predict this rise and to allow for it in workload allocation. It is the exceptional reviews which will present an unpredictable rise in work and, by their very nature, probably involve the care manager in more work, because their role will not only be to set up the review system, but also to offer support to those involved in a situation which has suddenly become volatile.

The scenario in which a care manager has to intervene suddenly and undertake direct work in situations where they have previously had a monitoring function while others have delivered services introduces a further aspect of workload management in care management. A simple numbers calculation would not suffice because, while there would be involvement of the care manager for the purpose of review, the person delivering the services might well continue contact with the client.

The issue here is one of double counting. Commonly in workload management terms double counting means that the worker is undertaking two (or more) tasks simultaneously and is allocated a weighting for each. An example of this in current practice is when a weighting is given for being duty officer but the worker is able to see his or her own clients, for which s/he also receives a weighting. In care management a different form of double counting will occur when a particular case is claimed as workload by more than one worker. It may be that in some cases a worker appointed as care manager will come from a different agency to that of the person directly providing the service and that parity of workloads is not an issue. However it could be that a number of workers from the same agency could be involved as, for example, care manager, broker and service provider.

In the case of the broker it may not be necessary to hand over the case, but there would need to be some acknowledgement of the contribution that the broker had made to the particular case. Similarly an acknowledgement of the care manager's overall responsibility for monitoring the case, together with a recognition of the direct work that might be at the point of, for example, review, needs to be identified in any allocation of weightings. At the same time such a system of workload allocation would need to give recognition to the input of the person who was delivering the service.

Much of the above discussion is based on two assumptions. The first is that different sets of tasks will be performed by different individual workers. To identify equitable measurements for such sets of tasks, while not necessarily an easy exercise, is simplified because the workload is held by an individual worker. However in earlier chapters we have acknowledged that there are a number of ways in which care management might be implemented. Acknowledgement of the tasks within care management and the appropriate allocation of weightings to them will be even more critical when workers perform a number of different functions within care management or, even more critically, when workers have a mixed caseload of cases requiring packages of care and those being offered social work service along traditional lines. The second assumption is that the *total* input into the process of care management needs to be monitored not only for the purposes of allocating workloads but also to ensure that all worker involvement, whatever the title, status or qualification of that worker, is acknowledged so that packages of care are properly costed.

A final point that needs to be given attention is the complicated question of what constitutes a care management task, and more particularly who decides what is appropriate for a worker to provide within a particular task. In our discussion of the management implications of care management we argued that, while care managers are themselves managers in their own right, they require a support system which among other things will take responsibility for monitoring and allocating workloads. A first requirement of this support system (which we have called service management) is to identify the tasks within care management and to ensure appropriate recognition of these within the workload allocation system. This identification and recognition will depend upon a supervision and monitoring process to ensure that workers do not attempt to do too much (or too little!) within a given task.

These are some underlying issues which need to be addressed when setting up a workload measurement system for care management. Such issues need to be addressed at the team level, as we identify in the next section, but could be assisted by work on a national scale along the lines of the National Probation Survey undertaken by the Home Office during 1990–91. In addition this work on measurement needs to be set into a fairly clear sequence of workload management issues related to the care management process.

Matching care and workload management

The sequence shown in Table 7.1 is an attempt to set side-by-side the components of a model of care management which we identified in the last chapter with the main features of workload management. The left-hand column traces the chronological path of care management. The right hand column identifies the corresponding workload management preoccupations.

This matching exercise demonstrates the extent to which a care management sequence depends on the availability of the tools of workload management. Care management rests on detailed information and the careful deployment of resources. Workload management first of all generates that information and then relates it to a range of necessary decision-making processes.

Measuring needs

In traditional social work practice the main purpose in measuring need is to get an idea of the anticipated amount of work required to provide a service. This knowledge then aids decisions about what resources can be allocated, and which social worker or other member of the team has the space to take on the client. At this stage the measurement is more correctly an estimate, made as part of the initial assessment, and subject to review as work with the client progresses. For that reason the tendency is to use a scale of categories or weightings into which the likely workload of a client's need is set (see, for example, Chapter 5 in Glastonbury, Bradley and Orme, 1987).

The role of needs measurement in care management is more substantial. The element of workload monitoring

Table 7.1

Care management	Workload management
Client needs focus	Identify overall needs level coming within remit of agency; this is the potential total workload.
Recording and tracking	Monitoring previous activity with clients
Assessment	Specification of needs at individual client level
Advocacy	Workload implications, e.g. if advocates are to be offered training, or funds paid to an advocacy group
Choosing a care manager	Care management type (i.e. specialist, with or without team co-ordination role, with non-care management duties) and consequent measurement of task; care management workload ceiling and overall workload ceiling setting
Planning the care package	Information (perhaps a catalogue) detailing cost and quality of available services. Immediate cost projections of a range of possible care packages; where services can be obtained, and availability of staff (i.e. task measurement and ceiling for those staff)
Devolution and resource flexibility	Division of funding responsibility; budgetary role at different hierarchical levels, and its co-ordination
Resource raising and brokerage	Cost/workload of broker; projection of income from external sources, or provision of free/subsidised services; impact on previous costing and measurements
Implementing the care package	Information relevant to purchasing decisions
The care package in action	Ongoing cost and workload impact; monitoring and quality control, including evaluation of services purchased

remains, but the focus moves more to the purchaser–provider relationship. Both sides require as accurate an assessment of the cost of service provision (including staff time) as possible because of the decisions they have to make in the process of contracting for services. It is impossible to operate this feature of care management without the ability to cost services for each individual client, or for a jointly contracted group of clients. Hence workload measurement is vital, and no care manager can afford to be unaware of service costs.

In practical terms there is a strong argument for an agency to invest in an initial workload audit and to use this as the basis for establishing baseline costs for services. In effect this would involve a study, whether national or local, similar to that undertaken in the probation service (Home Office, 1989) and designed to produce the equivalent of a catalogue of service costs. Running in parallel, service providers would develop their own catalogue of services on offer, with the prices to be charged. Once this infrastructure is in place, as it already is in the commercial market, the longer-term task becomes easier. The catalogues are updated from time to time, and local care managers have a baseline to work from, rather than having to calculate from basics for each client. Obviously local managers will have to make adjustments for local circumstances, but can do so with the knowledge of overview measurements. The NHS has already moved some way along the route to a purchaser–provider arrangement and the absence of an overall workload audit has shown up huge variations in locally stated prices. Without getting into the political argument about the desirability of encouraging price competition between local units, it has to be asserted that competitiveness and cost-effectiveness can only function well in the longer term if accurate costing can be produced.

Workload ceilings

There are long-established routes to setting workload ceilings outside the framework of a workload management system.

Custom and precedent are important. They tell us the approximate size of caseloads in different sorts of setting, for probation officers, child care workers, education welfare officers and others. They also tell us something about what proportions of a given caseload are likely at any given moment to be 'active', as opposed to those which are, albeit temporarily, dormant. Nevertheless this is a fundamentally flawed approach. It covers caseloads, but not the more relevant concept of workload, so it penalises those who make a contribution to the team and the agency in ways that are not directly client-related. More fundamentally, however, it offers minimal protection to staff, because in the last resort the size of a caseload is as high as the front line member of staff can be persuaded, cajoled or pressured into taking. Custom and precedent give a rough idea of average caseloads, not a realistic ceiling for the particular worker, in the particular circumstances s/he is experiencing.

Workload management systems function on total workloads, not just caseloads, and they allocate weightings for tasks, whether these weightings take the form of some kind of numerical score or a 'time for the job'. We have already explored some of the intricacies of allocating weightings to the tasks of care management, but a further requirement for the purpose of setting ceilings is that they relate to the contracted working week and what can be encompassed within it. They may, almost certainly will, acknowledge that emergencies arise which have to be handled despite workload implications, but the basic system ensures that in the long run a worker is not exploited in his or her terms of service.

The calculations possible within workload management allow some projection to be made of the time demands of commitments and the proportions of the working week they are expected to absorb. This in turn permits current and anticipated surplus capacity to be identified, so that whoever is responsible for work allocation can determine where it can be best placed. If there is no capacity to handle new work, then the system triggers mechanisms for checking the priority of new demands against those already in workloads. Hence, at times of high pressure, it draws attention to the lowest priority tasks, which become the focus for rationing. Such a system has distinct advantages for the practice of care management, provided it is suitably modified. The weakness of current workload management is that it is staff-focused. That is to say, the system seeks to handle only the allocation of tasks to members of staff and to relate those tasks to staff working capacity, the number of working hours they have available. Under care management the principle of measuring needs and servicing resources remains, but the definition of resources has to be widened from a limited focus on staff to the incorporation of all resources; that is, staff time, directly provided internal facilities and the purchasing capacity of funds to buy services. A workload management system for care and service managers must therefore have a clear view of the ceiling of all resources, and operationally it must offer three elements: (1) the total projected resource cost of any care package; (2) the priority rating of each element in that package; and (3) how that costing relates to current resource capacities. Note that the language has now changed a little, so that we now refer to the 'costs' of the package, rather than the weighting or the time needed. This recognises the move towards a more explicitly budgetary approach to measurement, but it still encompasses staff time, now in the form of the price to be paid, say, for the required number of hours of a social workers involvement.

A further modification concerns the way the system functions. Some early workload management systems, like the National Institute's case review system (Goldberg and Warburton, 1979), were criticised because of the time they took to administer. They added significantly to the overall workload. The previous paragraphs have suggested that a still more demanding form of workload measurement and management will be needed for care management. If it is to function in an acceptable way it will have to be automated, in effect computerised. At certain stages in the care management process it becomes necessary for vital resource information to be made immediately available. This is not the position at the point of assessment, but becomes so once the care packaging process begins. Care managers need to be able to ask 'What if . . .' questions. What will this care package cost, this week, next month, next financial year? What if a social work assistant is substituted for a level three social worker? What if case conferences are replaced by telephone contacts?

What is it going to cost?

At all stages of care packaging, from initial ideas through to the final commitment of services, it is vital to know the cost. In an overall agency sense this is literally the cash cost, the sum which will appear as a debit in the agency's annual accounts. At a more localised level, for the care manager, the cost has many components. There will be internal staff time and the price to be paid for externally contracted workers; service resources such as spaces in day or residential care; aids and adaptations, and many other items which are a direct part of the care package.

In addition there are infrastructural or overhead costs to be noted, including travel expenses, clerical support, heating, lighting, furnishing and cleaning, office space, and the care manager's own time. Against this can be set any income which is expected to arise, whether from client payments or from other sources. It is difficult to be precise about exactly what goes into a care package costing, because the context can be so varied. At one end of the spectrum, care management may operate in a setting which is, in effect, a fully devolved cost centre, responsible for its own budget. In this case all costs have to be met, including the sort of overhead examples given above. At the other end, care management may be a minor part of an agency's activity, so only the direct costs of care provision have to be worked out.

Important political decisions have to be made about the

extent of commitment to care management, and about the extent of devolution of resource responsibilities. These in turn will determine the coverage of the workload management facilities. One consideration will be the type of care manager model which is adopted, given that the commitment to care management can in itself become a significant resource issue. The focus to date has been on tasks connected with providing a service to clients and managing that provision. This is clearly the core role of the care manager, but there are other features to be taken into account. We have viewed care management as a team activity, very likely to involve staff from a variety of disciplines. Hence the task of team co-ordination comes into the reckoning, the job which is currently undertaken by someone designated or acting as key worker. There are also the demands of handling a mixed workload, partly care managed, partly using more established approaches. Again there are concerns of time which must be allowed to enable staff to develop and retain the capability to cope with such diversity.

At their core these points are reasserting the importance in workload management of viewing the total workload, not the more limited caseload. In this instance it is tempting to equate the care management load with the total workload, thus ignoring other items such as co-ordinating service teamwork for each client or acknowledging different approaches to service delivery, training, supervising students, keeping in touch with new developments, trying out new ideas, reviewing professional standards, and participating in wider agency activities. It is vital to avoid viewing the total costs of care management as solely those focused on the care package. If we fall into that trap then these other essential parts of the professional role will be elbowed out.

Priorities and rationing

The feature of workload management which is most fully developed in many agencies is the system for reducing the overall volume of need to the level which can be supported by existing resources. This is a two-pronged approach. First of all a priority rating is established, so that all current and new work can be given its place in a hierarchy of priority. Then a process of rationing takes place to filter out lower priority needs and ensure that limited resources are devoted to higher priority tasks. Under care management these two activities might be quite complex and multi-phased. Priorities can be generated at several stages in the assessment process, as a more detailed view of the client's needs develop. Rationing can be linked to the stages of assessment, so that clearly low priority needs are taken out before resources are committed to a more thorough assessment. The rationing system itself can have several routes, including passing clients to other agencies, giving them information and some advice on self-help, putting them on a waiting list, or just letting things stand in the hope (sometimes justified) that the need will go away.

Much of this will be familiar to personal social services staff, especially those in area offices. In care management the approach will have to be modified to observe the split between assessment and resource allocation. Under the sort of approach outlined above, the assessment process is influenced throughout by the view of the priority given to the needs being assessed, and therefore the chances of resources being allocated. Without wanting to suggest that the professional task of assessment is contaminated by awareness of the scale and range of resources, and of the rationing system in operation, it is clear that they are inextricably mixed in the overall procedures in current use. This may, as *Caring for People* (Department of Health, 1989) suggests, inhibit the creativity of service staff: at the same time it does allow a phased and sensitive approach to rationing. The separation of assessment from decisions about services will force a review of the way priority and rationing systems are to be applied. Undoubtedly an assessment process which is not tempered by a realistic idea of what the client is likely to get at the end of the line risks raising their expectations unnecessarily. The operation of rationing will have to take this into account. A supporter of care management might argue, with good sense, that the current amount of time spent on restricting service could be better employed searching out new forms of help, so making a rationing system less necessary. A sceptic will retort, also with good sense, that bricks are not made without straw, and that the need for rationing will depend on the level of resources society makes available to help those in need.

Summary

In this chapter we have brought together care and workload management and, in doing so, have identified the particular issues for constructing a workload measurement scheme for care management. The diversity of tasks to be identified in a workload, the measurement of individual tasks and the double counting of activities are examples of the complexity of such a process. It is apparent that much more needs to be undertaken in this area, but that this work is critical because in care management measurement of worker involvement directly equates to cost of the service.These measurement issues have to be incorporated into a workload management scheme and we have sought to give clarification to this by building on the model of care management presented in the last chapter and identifying the workload issues corresponding to each stage.

Conclusion

At the outset of this book we acknowledged that care management in community care, while building upon earlier policy and practice initiatives, brought with it the potential to change radically the face of social work. We have argued that, if care management does bring the opportunity for change and innovation, the implications for social workers must be considered. To do this, it is necessary to identify how the advantages and benefits of care management can reflect, and become enshrined in, good social work practice.

In the last two chapters we have provided a summary of what we feel are the essential processes within care management. In doing this we have concentrated on ways in which the social work profession will have to organise itself and provide a management structure to enable the essential values of social work to be incorporated into care management. We have argued that care management, while not being a new social work method (that is, a separate and different set of skills or actions) is, nevertheless, a means of intervention, a way of organising service delivery which can incorporate diverse methods and can be provided by a variety of individuals or organisations. There exist within this variety both the benefits and the risks of care management. The risks are that, with the possibility of a mixed economy of service provision, an element of competition will emerge. Provider agencies will attempt to win over consumers by

174

offering attractive services at economy prices. Purchasers, whether they be carers or people in need, will be required to choose on the basis of little information. Social services departments, who can be purchasers and providers, could become positively schizophrenic in an attempt to be all things to all people. Alternatively, the large organisations such as social services departments and health authorities could work to maintain a monopoly of the services, and thus deny consumers and carers of the best elements of care management the opportunity for choice. The benefits are that care management can provide the opportunity for organisations, public, voluntary and independent, to work together to ensure the widest possible choice for consumers, directly related to identified need.

The decision about collaboration or co-operation will be taken at the executive level of organisations such as social services departments. Care planning can be a glossy public relations exercise designed to quell the opposition, or it can be a genuine attempt to liaise with the community at all levels. However individual workers will also hold some responsibility. It is this tension which will have to be managed.

In putting care management into context we have identified other policy and practice initiatives that had similar potential, but have had mixed outcomes. It is our contention that those which had impact invariably made a link between practice and organisation and management. For example, the reorganisation of local authority social service departments along the lines recommended by the Seebohm Report (1968) enabled social workers to work to smaller geographical units. Hence there were boundaries to the work and the task seemed manageable. Further this reorganisation was supported by an increase in resources. A second example, that of task-centred casework (Reid and Epstein, 1972), illustrates how organisational structures can be linked to practice initiatives. The development of intake teams facilitated effective assessments and focused client work. Again this enabled social workers to control the work that they undertook, even if on this occasion there was an acknowledgement of the need to ration resources.

In many ways care management has some features of both the above. On the one hand it involves identifying client need and acknowledging resources available. The nub of the process is in the assessment. It therefore has close links with task centred work. On the other hand it involves acknowledging, as the Seebohm Report did, that social workers are very much agents within the community, and that service delivery must be organised/managed to identify both the needs within a community and the potential to meet those needs. Care management, however, goes further than both, linking the critical task of assessing need with the right of the person being assessed to contribute to that assessment, and to be involved in decisions about the services to be delivered. It is not concerned with rationing social worker time to those who are most likely to benefit from it, but with widening the potential sources from which the identified needs can be met, and providing a choice. In this way it embodies social work principles but widens the resources.

An essential ingredient of care management, task-centred work and the Seebohm reorganisation is that they all enable front line staff to work closely with those who are identified as having the need. This has implications both for the nature of the services which are provided and for their organisation. The front line worker identifies the needs and, ideally, resources are identified and services provided to meet them. However within this process the systems which are created to make the provision are also influenced by the workers. Hence generic area-based teams arose out of Seebohm, intake teams out of task-centred work. What sort of organisation of social services will arise out of care management?

The possibilities are manifold. For example, the emphasis on assessment links with a well-established skill and social workers could identify themselves as the general practitioners of social work provision, spending their time producing assessments which are then acted upon by others. Such an arrangement requires expertise in the process of performing an assessment but, if the organisation is further refined, assessment might be linked to particular groups of people, enabling the front line worker to develop an expertise in, for example, assessment of elderly people or those with mental health problems. Those workers who are not centrally involved in assessments would become involved in service provision.

This focused way of working will not, however, meet the needs of all currently employed as front line social workers, some of whom enjoy working over time with people, counselling, enabling and supporting. The opportunity to work in these ways does not disappear with care management; they can be critical factors in helping an individual with physical disabilities or learning difficulties, for example, to remain in the community. However the scope is widened. Attention has to be given to more than the repertoire of services currently available. Flair and imagination can be used to identify ways of meeting the need of, for example, companionship, help with getting in and out of bed or dealing with feelings of despair and anger. These can come from organisations other than the statutory social service departments. The private and independent sectors are being encouraged to become the providers of services which will be purchased by social service departments, care managers as their agents, or by individual consumers. However front line workers can also offer such intervention by being part of service provision, using specialist skills to focus on particular aspects of the situation, providing expert help. This could be done in an individual capacity or by a group of workers who share a common interest or set of skills forming consortia of service providers. A social service department would then have the option of contracting the necessary services from a variety of sources, including the specialists among their own staff. The benefit of purchasing from existing qualified staff is that the quality is tried and tested, and within the managerial control of social services.

It is when considering the range of resources that the individual worker can influence the outcomes of care management. It may be safe to choose consistently those services provided by colleagues within the social services departments, but it may not lead to innovative service provision. The significant issue is the need to have confidence in the management of the service delivery, the quality and the frequency of the intervention.

It is an awesome prospect to be responsible for the assessment of the individual, the identification of the resources and the provision of the resources. But in many ways social workers have been carrying such responsibilities for some time in individual cases. The benefits of care management, as we stated at the outset of this book, are that it involves the management of the care, not the case. As such it allows the individual worker autonomy within her/his own sphere of involvement but also demands that the management systems are in place to offer support to *all* involved in the process of offering care. Accountability is in the first instance to the person receiving the care but this can be mediated through the care manager and has to be overseen by the service manager. In many ways, if properly managed, care management can offer the protection of shared decision making.

But the key is in the notion of what proper management involves. Traditionally the management of community care has identified resources primarily as budgets and plant. This has led to calculations of need being made on day centre occupancy rates, home carers' hours or the cost of providing telephones. The balancing of the equation comes when those figures are matched against the cost of providing a place in a residential establishment. In care management this equation is still the crucial one, but the calculations that are done on the one side, what is needed to keep the person in the community, are being extended. Because the care package finally arrived at may not involve social workers from statutory social services and the setting up of the potential for provision will have involved a variety of resources, including worker time, a proper accounting of *all* input of services should be kept. This could include cash, the cost of providing transport or the time of the individual providing a service. To this end we have argued that at the outset a proper workload measurement system has to be in operation so that the distribution of tasks can be monitored and the total input recognised. A true monitoring of tasks and acknowledgement of input demands co-operation of the potential service providers rather than competition between them.

Only if a proper workload measurement system is in place can the tasks be managed to ensure job satisfaction for front line workers and to guarantee that people in need will not suffer by being denied the services of trained and experienced personnel. Care management provides the potential to manage the resources, but only if care management itself is properly managed will the necessary benefits accrue to the individual in need and social work as a profession survive.

Bibliography

Allan, G. (1983) 'Informal networks of care: issues raised by Barclay', *British Journal of Social Work*, no. 13, pp. 417–34.

Allen, I. (ed.) (1990) *Care Managers and Case Management*, London, Policy Studies Institute.

Audit Commission (1986) *Making a Reality of Community Care*, London, HMSO.

Bamford, T. (1982) *Managing Social Work*, London, Tavistock.

Bamford, T. (1990) *The Future of Social Work*, London, Macmillan.

Barclay, P. M. (1982) *Social Workers: their Role and Tasks*, London, Bedford Square Press.

Barr, H. (1971) *Volunteers in Prison After Care*, National Institute of Social Services Library No. 20, London, Allen and Unwin.

BASW (1977) *The Social Work Task*, Birmingham, British Association of Social Workers.

Beardshaw, V. (1990) 'Clearing the Mystery', *Community Care*, 28 June.

Biestek, F. (1961) *The Casework Relationship*, London, Allen and Unwin.

Bottoms, A. and McWilliams, W. (1979) 'A Non-treatment Paradigm for Probation', *British Journal of Social Work*, no. 9, pp. 159–202.

Brearley, C. P. (1982) *Risk and Social Work*, London, Routledge and Kegan Paul.

Brewer, C. and Lait, J. (1980) *Can Social Work Survive?* London, Temple Smith.

Brook, E. and Davis, A. (eds) (1985) *Women, the Family and Social Work*, London, Tavistock.

Caragonne, P. (1980) 'A Comparison of Case Management Work Activity Within the Texas Department of Mental Health and Mental Retardation', *Report for Texas Department of Mental Health and Mental Retardation*, April.

Carlyle, T. (1795–1881) *Chartism*.

Central Council of Education and Training (1989) *Multidisciplinary Teamwork: Models of Good Practice*, London, CCETSW.

Challis, D. and Davies, B. (1986) *Case Management and Community Care*, 1st edn, Aldershot, Gower.

Challis, D. and Davies, B. (1989) *Case Management and Community Care*, 2nd edn, Aldershot, Gower.

Commission for Racial Equality (1989) *Racial Equality in Social Services Departments: A Survey of Equal Opportunity Policies*, London, CRE.

Commission for Racial Equality (1990a) *Community Care and Ethnic Minority Communities: The Race Dimension*, London, CRE.

Commission for Racial Equality (1990b) *Response to 'Caring for People' Draft Guidance Circulars*, London, CRE.

Cooper, J. (1989) 'From Casework to Community Care', *British Journal of Social Work*, no. 19, pp. 177–88.

Corrigan, P. and Leonard, P. (1978) *Social Work Practice under Capitalism*, London, Macmillan.

Coulshed, V. (1988) *Social Work Practice: An Introduction*, London, Macmillan.

Coulshed, V. (1990) *Management in Social Work*, London, Macmillan.

Curnock, K. and Hardiker, P. (1979) *Towards a Practice Theory: Skills and Methods in Social Assessment*, London, Routledge and Kegan Paul.

Davies, M. (1981) *The Essential Social Worker: A Guide to Positive Practice*, Aldershot, Gower.

Davy, J. S. (1905–9) *Royal Commission on the Poor Law*.

Department of Health (1988) *Protecting Children: A Guide for Social Workers undertaking a Comprehensive Assessment*, London, HMSO.

Department of Health (1989) *Caring for People: Community Care in the Next Decade and Beyond*, Cmnd 849, London, HMSO.

Department of Health (1990) *Community Care in the Next Decade and Beyond. Policy Guidance*, London, HMSO.

Department of Health (1991a) *Purchase of Service: Practice Guidance and Practice Material for Social Services and Other Agencies*, London, HMSO.

Department of Health (1991b) *Assessment Systems and Community Care*, London, HMSO.

Department of Health (1992) *Hear Me, See Me. The report of the Beverley Lewis Inquiry*, London, HMSO.

Dominelli, L. (1988) *Anti-Racist Social Work: What Can White People Do?*, London, Macmillan.

Douglas, T. (1983) *Groups: Understanding people gathered together*, London, Tavistock.

Ely, P. and Denny, D. (1987) *Social Work in a Multi-Racial Society*, Aldershot, Gower.

Forbes, I. (1989) 'Unequal Partners: The Implementation of Equal Opportunities Policies in Western Europe', *Public Administration*, vol. 67, no. 1, pp. 19–38.

Finch, J. and Groves, D. (eds) (1983) *A Labour of Love: Women, Work and Caring*, London, Routledge and Kegan Paul.

Glastonbury, B. and Orme, J. (1990) 'Commentary on 1990 Care Plans', Hampshire Social Services, unpublished.

Glastonbury, B., Bradley, R. and Orme, J. (1987) *Managing People in the Personal Social Services*, Chichester: Wiley.

Goldberg, E. M. and Warburton, R. W. (1979) *Ends and Means in Social Work*, London, Allen and Unwin.

Gregory, J. (1987) *Sex, Race and the Law. Legislating for Equality*, London, Sage.

Griffiths Report (1988), *Community Care: Agenda for Action*, London, HMSO.

Hadley, R. and Hatch, S. (1981) *Social Welfare and the Failure of the State*, London, Allen and Unwin.

Hadley, R. and McGrath, M. (1984) *When Services Are Local: the Normanton Experience*, London, Allen and Unwin.

Hadley, R. and Young, K. (1990) *Creating a Responsive Public Service*, Brighton, Harvester Wheatsheaf.

Haines, J. (1975) *Skills and Methods in Social Work*, London, Constable.

Hanmer, J. and Statham, D. (1988) *Women and Social Work: Towards a Woman-Centred Practice*, London, Macmillan.

Home Office (1984) *Statement of National Objectives and Priorities for the Probation Service*, London, HMSO.

Home Office (1986) *Social Enquiry Reports*, Home Office Circular No. 92.

Home Office (1989) *Resource Management Information Systems*, Stage 3a, June, London, HMSO.

Home Office (1990) *Supervision and Punishment in the Community: A framework for action*, Cmnd 966, London, HMSO.

Horne, M. (1987) *Values in Social Work*, Aldershot, Wildwood House.

Hunter, D. J. (ed.) (1988) *Bridging the Gap: case management and advocacy for people with physical handicaps*, King Edward's Hospital.

NALGO (1989) *Social Work in Crisis: A Study of Conditions in Six Local Authorities*, London, NALGO.

NAPO (1979) *Probation Service Workload Measure – Revised Version*, London, National Association of Probation Officers.

Orme, J. (1988) 'Can Workloads be Measured?', *Probation Journal*, 35.2, pp. 57–9.

Orme, J. (1991) 'Research into the task of preparing a social inquiry report', National Association of Probation Officers, unpublished.

Parsloe, P. and Stevenson, O. (1978) *Social Service Teams: the Practitioners' View*, London, HMSO.

Pelletier, S. (1983) 'Developmental Disabilities Programmes', in C. Sanborn (ed.) *Mental Health Services*, New York, Haworth Press.

Piachaud, D. (1991) 'Revitalising Social Policy', *Political Quarterly*, vol. 62, no. 2, pp. 204-24.

Pincus, A. and Minahan, A. (1973) *Social Work Practice: Model and Method*, Ithaca, Illinois, Peacock.

Pitkeathley, J. (1990) 'Painful conflicts', *Community Care*, 22 February.

Plant, R. (1970) *Social and Moral Theory in Casework*, London, Routledge and Kegan Paul.

Priestley, P., Maguire, J., Flegg, D., Helmsley, V. and Welham, D. (1978) *Social Skills and Personal Problem Solving*, London, Tavistock.

Pritchard, C. (1985) *Maintaining Morale Through Staff Development and Training*, Social Work Monographs, Norwich, UEA.

Rees, S. (1978) *Social Work Face to Face*, London, Edward Arnold.

Reid, W. J. and Epstein, L. (1972) *Task-Centred Casework*, Columbia, Columbia University Press.

Renshaw, J. (1988) 'Care in the Community: Individual Care Planning and Case Management', *British Journal of Social Work*, no. 18, pp. 79–105.

Sainsbury, E. (1970) *Social Diagnosis in Casework*, London, Routledge and Kegan Paul.

Seebohm Report (1968) *Report of the Committee on Local Authority and Allied Personal Social Services*, Cmnd 3703, London, HMSO.

Sheldon, B. (1978) 'Theory and Practice in Social Work: a Re-examination of a Tenuous Relationship', *British Journal of Social Work*, no. 8, pp. 1–22.

Smale, G. and Tuson, G. (1990) 'Community Social Work: Foundations for the 1990s and Beyond', in G. Darvill and G. Smale (eds), *Partners in Empowerment: Networks and Motives*, London, NISW.

Social Services Inspectorate (1991a) *Purchase of Services: Practice Guidance and Practice Material for Social Service Departments and Other Agencies*, London, HMSO.

Social Services Inspectorate (1991b) *Assessment Systems and Community Care*, London, HMSO.

Steinberg, R. and Carter, G. W. (1983) *Case Management and the Elderly*, Lexington, Mass., Lexington Books.

Timms, N. and Timms, R. (1977) *Perspectives in Social Work*, London, Routledge and Kegan Paul.

Towle, C. (1965) *Common Human Needs*, USA, NASW.

Tutt, N. (1990) *Assuring Quality in Community Care*, Southampton, CEDR.

Ungerson, C. (1987) *Policy is Personal*, London, Tavistock.

Vickery, A. (1976) 'A Unitary Approach to Social Work with the Mentally Disordered', in R. Olsen (ed.), *Differential Approaches in Social Work*, Birmingham, British Association of Social Workers.

Vickery, A. (1977) *Caseload Management*, London, National Institute of Social Work Papers No. 5.

Webb, A. (1983) 'Strained Relations', in *The Concise Barclay: Digest and Commentary*, Birmingham, British Association of Social Workers.

Webb, A. and Wistow, G. (1987) *Social Work, Social Care and*

Social Planning: The Personal Social Services since Seebohm, Harlow, Longman.

Webb, B. and S. (1929) *English Poor Law History*, London, private subscription.

Wilson, E. (1980) 'Feminism and Social Work', in R. Bailey and M. Brake (eds), *Radical Social Work Practice*, London, Edward Arnold.

Glossary

This short glossary offers brief definitions and descriptions of terms used throughout the book in the discussion of care and workload management. Generally more detailed explanations are given within the text, but the reader may find the following list a useful point of reference.

Advocacy. The process of ensuring that the views, circumstances and needs of a member of the public are fully and effectively represented to service agencies. Advocacy is generally employed when the member of the public cannot adequately represent his or her own position.

Advocate. The person who carries out the advocacy task on behalf of another. In care management an advocate has an identified role and may be a relative or friend of a client, or someone specifically taken on to undertake advocacy.

Assessment. Assessment is a central feature of care management. It is a process in which a person's circumstances are fully analysed and her/his needs identified. A further feature of care management is that assessment is a self-contained process, carried out independently of the allocation of services.

Broker. As with an advocate, a broker is another potential member of the care management team. The broker is a person whose task is to identify possible service resources (for example, in the voluntary sector) and where necessary help to generate new resources. These resources can then be commissioned by the purchasing agency and be available when packages of care are constructed.

Budgetary devolution. As a generalisation it is traditional for the finances of a social services agency to be managed through centralised control and accountancy systems, with only small-scale resources available for use at the discretion of front line staff. A facet of the theory of care management is that more extensive control over finances (budgets) will need to be transferred (devolved) to operational units closer to the point at which direct service provision is handled.

Care management. The label given in the UK to the task of organising and overseeing the provision of a care package for a client who has been assessed, and whose needs are considered of sufficient priority to warrant the allocation of services. In North American literature the term *Case management* may be used instead.

Care manager. The member of agency staff whose job (wholly or partly) is care management. This person is likely to be a social worker, but may be a different agency employee (such as a home care organiser) or in certain circumstances could be a competent client managing her/his own care package.

Care package. Once a person's assessment is completed, there is a process of identifying whether that person's needs warrant services provision (matters like statutory responsibility and the availability of resources come in here) and if a high enough priority is agreed then appropriate services are sought. Within care management, services should be carefully planned, identified and established to meet the assessed needs of the client. Services set up in this way form the care package.

Care plan. A care plan covers the way a care package is initially designed (based on the assessment), the planned process for implementing the care package, and the arrangements for a review and evaluation.

Carer. In many circumstances, especially with elderly people, a client is looked after on a day-to-day basis by a carer. The existence of a large population of unpaid carers is fundamental to the survival of our current range of services. In care management the notion of informal carers becomes prominent. These can be either family members of the person needing the care, or volunteers recruited, usually on an unpaid basis, either directly or through a voluntary organisation. Formal carers are those who are employed by statutory and voluntary organisations. The carer should be recognised as an integral part of the assessment and care management processes, and as someone whose task of caring needs active agency support.

Case management. As mentioned (see *Care management* above), *case management* is sometimes used instead of *care management*. In some UK literature and agencies a case manager is a person who oversees a cluster of care management arrangements, perhaps all of those in a particular locality, or all of those carried out by a group of care managers. In this text we have generally used the term *service manager* to describe this role.

Commissioning. The theory of care management argues that, if the appropriate range of services cannot be found in order to establish a care package which meets assessed needs, then consideration should be given to the imaginative development of new provisions. The term *commissioning* refers to the processes of making the arrangements to develop a new provision and (for example, with a new building) taking over a new facility and making it operational.

Community care. Community care is the central platform of social policy upon which the personal social services operate. In this context it is commonly set alongside residential care, with the policy stating that where at all possible people's needs should be met in a community setting, rather than in a residential institution. At a more detailed level *community care* refers to the complex network of services and supports which enable people with needs or with a loss of independent functioning to continue to live in their own homes.

Complaints procedure. It is a requirement placed on all local authority social services departments that they have in place a procedure to deal fairly, effectively and promptly with complaints received from members of the public (clients, users, consumers, carers).

Consumer. Several labels are used to describe those who receive services. Traditionally in the personal social services they have been called *clients*, while the health services have referred to *patients.* In recent years the terms *user* and *consumer* have come into wider use, partly to reflect a growing interest in consumerist issues, and partly to reflect the language of commerce.

Consumerism. The philosophy which places strong emphasis on a person's right to self-determination, to make his or her own life decisions. In the personal social services a consumerist approach is one which seeks to assert a role for consumers (users, clients) both in general decision making and in decisions affecting each specific individual (consumer).

Contracting. Once a care package has been agreed, specified individuals or agencies have to be appointed to provide the relevant services. Within care management a contact is made between the agency providing the resources (see *purchaser* below) and those who will be directly responsible for providing services (see *provider* below). This is a technical process of establishing a legal contractual relationship. However, *contracting* also has a use in social work for the non-technical, non-legal forming of an agreement between a social worker and client covering agreed services and the range of responsibilities on both sides.

Demand. See *Need and demand* below.

Devolution. Part of the general theory of care management is that, for it to be effective, greater authority must rest at the front line of service provision than is traditional in a hierarchical agency. *Devolution* is used to describe the transfer of authority to appropriate low levels in the agency hierarchy. This may refer specifically to financial matters (see *Budgetary devolution* above) or more generally to the point in an agency hierarchy where client based decisions are taken.

Empowerment. Generally set within the context of consumerism, *empowerment* refers to the process by which clients (users, consumers) begin to take, or are helped to take, greater responsibility for their own lives and services.

Enabling. At its simplest level this is offering people support or making it easier for them to make and carry through their own decisions about their lives. However, within social work, the notion of *enabling* is part of the debate about the appropriate balance of 'providing services' and 'helping people to help themselves' (that is, enabling people).

Front line. In a social services agency there are staff who have direct face-to-face contact with clients, for example as part of assessment or the provision of services, and there are other staff with different tasks (such as administration, planning and overall agency management) who may have little or no direct contact with clients. The *front line* refers to those locations and agency staff groups who interact directly with clients, at the point of assessment and service delivery.

Front line manager. This is used to describe a person who is responsible for managing front line activities and/or front line staff groups.

Independent sector. Traditionally personal social services in the UK have been provided through public (governmental) agencies, generally organised and run by local authorities. There has been a role for the voluntary and private sectors, but a relatively small one. As part of its plan to develop community care outlined in *Caring for People* (Department of Health, 1989) anticipates the development of an independent sector of welfare provision (a combination of voluntary and private sectors) which can play a growing part in overall servicing. The issue is generally viewed as politically motivated, rather than an integral part of the theories of community care or care management.

Intake (duty). Both of these words are used colloquially within the personal social services to describe the arrangement an agency sets up to handle incoming referrals. Such referrals may come from another agency (for example, from the police or court), but commonly will arise when a member of the public comes to a local office seeking information, advice or help. *Intake* and *duty* describe different ways of receiving visitors and other forms of referral. *Intake* often refers to a small staff team who specialise in reception work, while *duty* is more often used when staff with wider job descriptions spend a period (a day per week, for example) on duty at the point of intake.

Key worker. It has long been recognised that meeting the needs of an individual client may require the involvement of a group of different service staff. So that such a group may operate effectively as a team, it has been a traditional practice to appoint one of them, often the social worker, to an overall co-ordinating role. This person is usually referred to as the key worker and, as our text suggests, there are many of the tasks carried out by the key worker in the new role of care manager.

Need and demand. Social theory distinguishes between the level of *need* for social services, in the sense of the proportion of population groups whose circumstances would warrant or make them eligible for services, and *demand* as expressed by those who come forward to seek service, or are referred through some other channel. A number of studies (especially in the field of welfare benefits) have drawn attention to the overall level of need, and the smaller scale of demand, with resulting concern about those who have needs (or are eligible for benefits) but do not come forward to receive them. In social work it is often assumed that demand falls well below need because many people find a solution to their problems through the help of friends, relatives, local networks and so forth. However it is also a cause of concern that some need (for example, in relation to child abuse or isolated very elderly people) is unrecognised and untreated.

Performance indicators. See *Quality measurement* below.

Purchaser/provider. Traditionally within the personal social services the agency which purchases services for its clients (that is, provides the budgetary resources) also directly provides the necessary services. At a subsidiary level only there has been some separation of the purchasing and providing roles, as in the way a statutory agency contracts with and funds a voluntary organisation to carry out certain tasks. Within the framework of new community care services (and indeed within the National Health Service) the argument has been made that greater efficiency will follow from a wider separation of the roles of *purchaser* and *provider*, even where both are part of the same employing agency.

Quality assurance. As with *Complaints procedure* above, local authority social services departments are required to have in place a formal means for assuring the acceptable quality of service provision. Many other agencies have followed suit. *Quality assurance* is widely viewed as being concerned with setting general standards and carrying out regular inspections. The role of central government inspectorates, like the Social Services Inspectorate of the Department of Health, should also be noted.

Quality measurement. Setting standards for an acceptable quality of service provision also involved establishing a process by which quality can be measured. Measures of both quality and quantity of service provision are taken into account in the development of *Performance indicators*, which are formal (increasingly nationally based) ways of shedding light on the effectiveness and efficiency of local services.

Resource generation. Part of the political agenda for new community care services is widely held to be the aim of either reducing the proportion of public funding which goes into social servicing or of supplementing public funding with new non-public resources. *Resource generation* is the task of seeking to identify new resources, and is commonly associated with the role of *broker*.

Self-management. Within the context of *Workload management* (see below) an important task is the way social workers and other front line staff handle their own workloads. This includes, for example, use of time, setting priorities and meeting deadlines. Workload management within an agency is seen as a combination of 'being managed' (by a manager) and managing oneself.

Service management. See *Case management* above. *Service management* is the task of overseeing and co-ordinating a cluster of care packages, perhaps all those in a particular locality, or all those being carried out by a group of care managers.

Service manager. This is the person responsible for service management, and in order to carry out that role he or she is likely to be found at or near the agency front line. In practice a service manager could be the personnel or line manager of care management staff, but this is an unlikely arrangement (see *Team manager* below).

Team manager. A locally based member of the agency who is the line manager of agency staff within that location, responsible for personnel and administrative arrangements, among other things. A local office may have several team managers (for example, for social workers or teams of clerical staff).

Teamwork. The process by which a group of people responsible for service provision co-ordinate their activities to provide a coherent service for each client, in line with the care package.

Value for money. This is the phrase used to focus on the quality and quantity of service which can be provided for a given input of resources. There are many other terms used within this particular discussion, such as *cost–benefit*, *cost-effectiveness* and *productivity*.

Vire. This verb is used as a technical term to describe the transfer of funds from one planned form of expenditure to another. For example, if the funds allocated for the provision of meals on wheels are underspent, but those for the provision of telephones to housebound people are overspent, then funds must be 'vired' from the meals on wheels budget to the telephone budget.

Workload/caseload. A workload is the total range of tasks carried by a member of agency staff (including such items as training), while a caseload is the number of cases or clients for whom the member of staff is responsible.

Workload management. This is the phrase used to describe the way in which the range of tasks carried by a social worker or other member of a social services or probation agency are co-ordinated, carried out to appropriate standards, monitored and reviewed.

Workload measurement. In order for workloads to be established which fit within the contracted working week of the employee, or in order to discover how much time and resource is needed for a particular task, a system of measuring work is needed. *Workload measurement* is not normally carried out in relation to each individual task, but through an attempt to identify the average amount of work involved in a particular category of task. An example of this in the probation service is the notional time ascribed to the task of preparing a social enquiry report for a court.

Author Index

Subject Index